Natural Hormone

Replacement
For Men and Women

How to Achieve Healthy Aging
2nd Edition

Neal Rouzier, M.D.

WorldLink Medical Publishing
Salt Lake City

The stories in this book are reflections of experiences by the author. Patients' names and personal information have been changed to protect their privacy. The recommendations, procedures and opinions in this book are those solely of the author and are not meant to replace the services of a trained health professional. All matters regarding your health require medical supervision. If you have preexisting conditions, you should consult with a doctor before practicing any of the procedures within these pages. Neither the author nor the publisher will be held liable or responsible for any loss, injury, or damage allegedly arising from any information or suggestion in this book.

Provera® is the registered trademark of Pfizer Inc.
Prempro® is the registered trademark of Wyeth Pharmaceuticals
Arimidex® is a trademark of the AstraZeneca group of companies
Synthroid® is the registered trademark of Abbott Laboratories
Levoxyl® is a registered trademark of King Pharmaceuticals Research and Development, Inc.
Armour® Thyroid is the registered trademark of Forest Laboratories, Inc.
Rozerem™ is a trademark of Takeda Pharmaceutical Company

Printed and bound in the United States.

WorldLink Medical Publishing
801-294-1330

Library of Congress Cataloging-in-Publication Data
ISBN 0-9710007-3-5

For orders other than by individual consumers, WorldLink
Medical Publishing offers a discount on the purchase of ten or
more books. For further details, please write to:
books@mqrx.com or 669 West 900 North, North Salt Lake
City, Utah, 84054, ATTN: Book Sales.

Books can be ordered online at www.mqrx.com or through
www.amazon.com.

Acknowledgements

To my wife, Carolyn, who makes the clinics and my endeavors in this field a reality. She is my researcher, typist, proofreader, nurse, office manager, organizer, personal secretary, housekeeper, chef, gardener, and best friend.

To Jacque Butler, and MedQuest Pharmacy, whose support and generosity brought this book out of the wood work.

To Cherie Constance, Bridgette Redman and Kyle Riley for their research and editing skills that made my words come alive.

To my patients, true examples of healthy aging, who brought life and personality to this book.

To medical research teams that bring credence and significance to the field of preventive medicine.

But most of all, I dedicate this book to the many doctors who refuse to explore the medical field outside their box. I write this book specifically for you and your patients in hopes that this book will be a catalyst for change, and that patients everywhere will receive the type of medical care worthy of being called quality preventive medicine.

"A solid work that piques the curiosity and encourages deeper investigation. Most admirably, it steers clear of vanity, and onto a course designed to promote a healthy, high-quality life."

"[Rouzier] approaches the issue from two angles, arguing that preventive hormonal therapy can stem deterioration (but not restore what has been lost), and that specifically fashioned, bio identical hormones are the only ones worth taking because they are fabricated to couple with an individual's receptors."

-- Kirkus Discoveries

"Each hormone and its use are thoroughly discussed to include patients' symptoms, benefits and suggested dosages. Patients' stories are included to support the research. The author has included a bibliography in the back of the book to indicate medical sources..."

"Easy to follow guide in layman's terms, this book is informative and educational. This reviewer was also entertained by the anecdotes from patients and researchers. Well worth a look by anyone concerned with aging, declining health and overall well-being..."

--AllBooks Review

"As an innovator and leader in the research, development and art of longevity medicine, Dr. Rouzier introduces new ways to get your youth back naturally. Taking certain natural hormones orally as well as taking natural estrogen and testosterone hormones would allow your body to heal (thus anti-age) and prevent wear and tear just like years before. Other lesser-known hormones that existed abundantly when we were young but diminish as we age are also introduced to the readers. *How to Achieve Healthy Aging...* introduces a new paradigm on preventing diseases and maintaining our youth. The down-to-earth explanations, impressive statistics and case studies are both insightful and encouraging.

How to Achieve Healthy Aging is definitely an invaluable contribution to modern medicine and society."

--BookReviewClub.com

"When it comes to medical decisions, a second opinion is usually advised. Dr. Rouzier is the third opinion we would all love to have. He provides information on what we need or might not need to help us make an informed decision."

Christine Summers
Host of Body Talk
Syndicated Health and Wellness Radio Show
Health Radio Network

Table of Contents

Forward   13
Introduction: My Story of Healthy Aging   17
    The Moment of Youth   18
    Supply and Demand   19
    Hormones: The Magic Bullet Program for Aging   22
    A Quick Word of Advice   26
    What You're Up Against   28
Are Hormones Beneficial or Harmful   31
DHEA: The Age Gauge   37
    Laid Up With Colds?   42
    Stress: The Second Pillar of Age   43
    Cancer: The Rooted Disease   46
    A Hearty Hormone   47
    Adagio for Looking Good and Feeling Good   49
    Where to Start   51
Estrogen: The Genesis of Hormone Replacement   55
    The Women's Health Initiative (WHI)   59
    Not Just a Matter of Semantics   62
    Estrogen: The What's, How's, and Whys   64
    The Menopause Cure-All   66
    Osteoporosis: A Breakthrough for Healthy Bones   71
    Harnessing Heart Disease   74
    Brain Food   76
    The Estrogen Scare: Breast and Ovarian Cancer   78
    What Does This All Mean?   83
Progesterone: Estrogen's Natural Sidekick   85
    Ready to Get Off the Mood Swing?   89
    Matters of the Heart   91
    Bone Up   95
    Since I Don't Have a Uterus, My Doctor Says I Don't
        Need Progesterone   96
    Synthetic vs. Natural   98
    The Challenge   104

Estrogen, Progesterone and Cancer:
   What's the Real Story   107
Testosterone: Revitalize Every Aspect of Your Life   113
   Slipping Into Lower Gear   115
   Total vs. Free Testosterone—There is a Difference   117
   Balancing Act: The Testosterone-Estrogen Ratio   119
   The Ultimate Aphrodisiac   122
   Improving Your Emotional State   125
   Lose that Middle!   127
   Out With the Old, In With the New   129
   What it Really Means to Have a Good Heart   132
   The Smart Hormone   134
   Keeping the Prostate Under Control   136
   Estrogen and Progesterone in Men   139
   Fine-Tune Yourself for the Years to Come   144
Testosterone: the Women's Side of the Story   147
   Are You in the Mood?   151
   Building Bone with Hormones   155
   More Side Benefits of Testosterone for Women   157
   Testosterone: The Female Hormone   158
Thyroid: The Most Misunderstood Hormone   161
   Thyroid is an Essential Hormone   165
   Your Amazing Thyroid   167
   Why am I Always Cold?   170
   News to Cure the Blues   172
   Weak from Fatigue?   175
   Thyroid for the Heart?   176
   Thyroid and Your Hair   178
   My Levels are Normal, But I Feel Terrible   179
   What Thyroid Should I Be Taking?   182
   How to Be Heard   185
Melatonin: The Aging Loophole   187
   Nature's Little Pacemaker   190
   Sleep: Nature's Tonic   191
   Keeping our Immune System Strong   193
   Cancer - A Common Foe of Aging   196
   Is Melatonin for You?   197

Epilogue: Making the Choice for a Healthy Longevity   **199**
     Where We Stand Today   **201**
     Pharmacies of the Past, Reshaping the Future   **203**
     Are You Ready?   **205**
Bibliography – The Scientific Justification for Bio
     Identical Hormones   **207**
Biography – Neal Rouzier, M.D.   **245**

Forward
by Dr. Douglas Dedo

...our hormones keep us healthy and when restored to
optimal ranges, they keep us energetic and youthful...

—Dr. Neal Rouzier

The fountain of youth - a magical, elusive spring
Ponce de Leon searched for as an elixir for the aging process -
may be closer than we think. Dr. Neal Rouzier has written his
answer for the vagaries of aging by sharing with us his story
and how it forced him to expand his vision from mainstream
medicine to "preventive medicine".

As I write this forward I am torn between writing
from the perspective of a facial cosmetic surgeon, a natural
hormone replacement physician, or as a patient myself. As Dr.
Rouzier reached his early forties, he began his intellectual
pursuit of the benefits of natural hormone replacement
therapy. I too kept my eyes and ears open for the endless
possibilities in this exciting field of medicine.

In 1997, as I felt life escaping, I decided it was time to
begin my personal journey. Middle age symptoms increased
and my energy quickly declined. I felt as if my intellectual and
sexual function had bottomed out. I looked at this as the
"standard" of living for the next years of my life.

Just as Dr. Rouzier studied the peer-reviewed journals,
I too, voraciously studied everything I could get my hands on.
In *Natural Hormone Replacement for Men and Women: How to
Achieve Healthy Aging*, Dr. Rouzier makes it easy for the
interested patient to read and understand the effects of each
hormone on the aging process.

Furthermore, Dr. Rouzier does not quote "junk science". He has an incredible bibliography of peer-reviewed journals that would satisfy a medical school professor or physician looking to educate themselves in this field. I strongly encourage patients to read this book and make their own choices about the aging process. I then ask each patient to share this book with their physician.

I can attest to the difference it has made in my own life. After two months on the program I lost my gut, my energy levels were back to normal and sexually I was quite pleased. Interestingly, my patients began to comment on my skin and overall appearance. They expressed their personal need to feel and look better. Naturally this would lead into a discussion on HRT. They were frustrated by being told "it's the aging process; just learn to live with it." I soon began to incorporate longevity medicine in my own practice. Many of the testimonies in this book could have come from my own patients.

I personally have found longevity and preventive medicine to be a natural extension of cosmetic surgery. Patients find they can surgically reverse the effects of gravity and aging through face-lifts, eyelifts and liposuction. These procedures certainly make them look better, but cannot halt the internal aging process. When I prescribe HRT to a patient before surgery, they heal faster and feel better post-operatively. If the patient continues the natural hormone supplements post-operatively, two wonderful things happen. First, they will probably never need a second tuck or facelift. Second, they will begin to feel good with increased energy, libido, skin texture, muscle-to-fat distribution and improved mental clarity. Most of all, I give my surgical patients a choice in how they age after their cosmetic surgery!

For those who are interested in an increased quality of life, I ask them to read *Natural Hormone Replacement for Men and Women*. This book answers their questions and makes my job of communicating with their physician much easier.

Throughout my lectures on how to incorporate natural hormone replacement into a surgical practice, I conclude with the following to my fellow facial and cosmetic surgeons: It is not IF you will incorporate HRT in your practice but WHEN. As you age, you will demand it for yourself and subsequently for your patients.

Introduction:
My Story of Healthy Aging

The reasons for some animals being long-lived and others short-lived, and in a word, causes of the length and brevity of life calls for investigation.
—Aristotle, "The Longevity and Shortness of Life"

Throughout this book I will share my own personal rejuvenation stories and the stories of my patients. After embarking on my personal hormone replacement journey, aging became scarcely noticeable.

Prior to becoming an impassioned believer in natural hormone replacement, I sat on a firm seat in the conventional medicine camp. I followed the orthodox beliefs of conservative medicine. By doing this, I assumed I was serving the common good of each patient. In the emergency room, I treated situations to the best of my ability, some very far from being 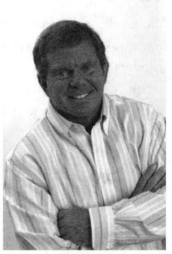 treatable. Treating the disease rather than the patient was considered the charge of a "good" doctor. I knew how to treat a cardiac arrest and a stroke, yet I had no idea how to prevent these events from happening. Preventive medicine seemed an ideal rather than a reality — certainly there was a lot to learn.

My introduction to preventive medicine was spurred by selfishness. As I turned forty-three, the effects of aging crept into my daily activities. I felt lethargic and my body immediately responded to the decline. I gained weight, my skin and hair texture lost their healthy glow. Most of all, I no longer had the drive to continue my disciplined exercise regimen. When I wanted to exercise, I just couldn't do it because I had so much joint pain. My passion for racing cars began to wane. With this new reality check, I realized I was just getting old. Anxiety hit and I spiraled into that mid-life crisis. Instead of giving in, I embraced more complex and unconventional views of aging. The bogus products and programs promising the magic of restoring youth were overwhelming. Along with the promises came bad science. Marketing companies focused on vulnerable patients who urgently sought to reverse age-related diseases and physical deterioration. I found myself frustrated with each of these deceptive promises. My personal goal was to feel good enough to find my passion and drive one more time. Nothing seemed to hold any real promise.

The Moment of Youth

Among the magical elusive fountains of youth, I stumbled upon natural hormone replacement therapy. These treatment modalities had clinical backup from peer-reviewed journals. Natural Hormone Replacement was rapidly gaining respect and notoriety. It not only appeared to work, but went above and beyond the expectations of doctors and scientists. After much investigation and consideration, my personal treatment program with this new therapy began. My success was immediate and led me to implement this new protocol of optimal hormone replacement therapy into my practice.

From a tired aging man, I quickly became a vigorous entrepreneur of hormone replacement therapy. My workload picked up the pace. With endless energy I returned to the gym for my daily work out. My sleep was unbelievable. Most of all, my wife liked me much, much better after only three months of my program. This was a "born-again" experience, with the source of my redemption being bio identical hormones. I had stumbled upon the answer to painful aging, recognizing that optimal health was truly what the term "preventive medicine" was all about.

This discovery forced me to quickly change my traditional thoughts on medicine. I no longer regarded aging as a human condition, an inevitable lot in the deterioration of life. I realized aging was something we could alter and control. Joining the ranks of the minorities who treat aging with hormones, I could now promote well-being through natural hormone replacement therapy. What an awesome notion! We can now take measures to hinder the symptoms of growing older. This was something the whole world needed to know. With hormone replacement therapy, I felt alive again. Beyond feeling and function, HRT was protecting me from the deterioration of neurological, cardiovascular and musculoskeletal systems as expected with normal aging.

Supply and Demand

In spite of the daily ups and downs, humans strive to live to a ripe old age. Why is this? I've followed the pattern of older people in my practice over the years—bent over, frail, and suffering from age-related declines. Their fate is unappealing and nerve-wracking. Personally, I eat a healthy diet, exercise and have plans to live well beyond the normal life expectancy. Perhaps this is a facet of the human instinct, something comparable to survival of the fittest. Unfortunately, survival does not necessarily mean quality of life. The question isn't whether I want to live a long life, but whether I want to ambitiously live a long life full of vigor and vitality.

The most deceptive information we hear is "aging is normal." The decline (cognitive, physical, emotional) we experience is "normal" and we should just learn to live with it. We should just fall prey to osteoporosis, heart disease, Alzheimer's or cancer -- no one lives forever. More importantly, some say no one can prevent or improve this decline. As a doctor and a patient, this kind of apathy is frustrating. I'm excited to say that there *is* a silver lining. As I delved into the genre of this new research, I found that major, esteemed medical institutions felt the same way, and were researching hormones for their role in health and well-being. Hormones, it appeared, were the key to a longer, healthier life.

The endocrine system, comprised of glands which produce and send hormones to various areas of the body, regulate all essential functions of the human body, the most important of these being temperature, reproduction, growth,

> **I think it might be possible to modulate the key hormones growth hormone, thyroid hormone, insulin growth factor, and if we can modulate those in a healthy range—maintain our health but toward a level that can permit us to slow aging—I think it's possible to do it.**
>
> —*Marc Tatar (Longevity Scientist at Brown University).*

aging, and the immune system. It stands to reason that science's primary focus should be optimal health. Science is unraveling the aging code by analyzing each hormone's action and reaction. We now see that when hormones are at optimal levels, the body is healthy and in better physical condition. This ideal function of the body can falter with any change in hormones. Sleep, diet, and exercise influence our essential levels; however, by themselves, they do not delay the decline. Physical, emotional, and mental deterioration are also a direct reflection of the state of our hormones. Declining levels may cause an increase in disease and the physical deterioration we associate with aging. Research demonstrates that the only solution to alter this age-associated decline is through hormone supplementation. The desire for youth has created a rift in the medical and ethics community. Who are we to mess with Mother Nature? Who are we to doctor-up the natural sequence of human life: we are born, we get older, we deteriorate and we die. They will contend this kind of medicine is cosmetic and fueled more by narcissism than by the desire to live longer and better. You will see throughout this book, I will contest the definition of "normal." I will argue that conservative doctors and the ethicists do more harm than good. Optimal hormone therapy, or more correctly termed "preventive" medicine, is about more than just vanity; it is our health and quality of life.

In light of the criticism, there is a large demand among many people contemplating their demise while seeking to find the aging loophole. Forward-thinking doctors are now the supply to this demand. The clinically proven benefits of natural hormone replacement therapy cannot be ignored. While many physicians find themselves unfamiliar with this advance in medicine, the medical literature very adequately supports the concept and demonstrates the harmful effects of low hormone levels. It is obvious that optimal hormone replacement therapy improves the health and well-being of both men and women.

Hormones: The Magic Bullet Program for Aging

Before delving into the descriptions of our essential hormones, I would like to give you a brief taste of the sweet possibilities they offer an aging body. This overview will only wet your appetite as you begin your own quest for healthy aging. We live in an era which fortunately offers access to hormones. These options were not available to previous generations. They were simply left to suffer in silence. Science and medicine now offer you this opportune moment. I encourage you to seize it now.

DHEA: This is the most abundant hormone in the human body and has become a celebrity of the hormone regimen. Varying opinions either boost its reputation as a multifunctional, age-defying hormone or decry its status, saying it's more hype than reality. DHEA has been found to affect the body in its own right, but also by way of conversion into testosterone, estrogen, or progesterone. Clinical studies have revealed that DHEA has a profound effect on the immune system, sex drive, metabolism, and one's emotional stability. Its effect on the immune system via regulation of stress hormones and by its function as a powerful antioxidant illustrates one of its age-resisting capabilities. Other health-related benefits include its ability to alter cognitive decline, help the body cope with stress, and its healthy influence over the heart by way of cholesterol modulation. Unfortunately, these benefits decline with age. Proven studies keep DHEA in the news and in the interest of people who strive to remain healthy in their later years. As a quick side note, the FDA has shown signs of approval of DHEA as a drug to treat serious illnesses such as lupus and connective tissue disease.

Melatonin: This hormone is produced by the pineal gland, the gland some scientists believe to be the source of our body's aging. It controls the activities of virtually every cell in the body. Melatonin regulates the circadian rhythm as well as the deep stages of sleep. Within these deep stages of sleep the immune system is stimulated. In a January 1997 issue of the New England Journal of Medicine, melatonin was extolled as a powerful antioxidant, a potential anti-cancer agent, and a perfect candidate to put on the list of essential hormones. Studies using mice have shown the addition of melatonin can return 24-month old mice to their more youthful, active state. In light of the hundreds of studies showing melatonin can scavenge free radicals, fight cancer and induce youthful sleep patterns, it's a shoe-in for everyone's hormone regimen.

Estrogen: This is the genesis of hormone replacement therapy, and has been prescribed for more than 40 years for women suffering the symptoms of menopause. Because estrogen went above and beyond just staving off the bothersome symptoms of menopause, women opted to continue this therapy. Researchers began to explore the other therapeutic realms of estrogen. Physically speaking, women have seen favorable changes in muscle tone, wrinkles, hair texture, and libido. Medically speaking, study after study illustrates that estrogen should not be used as a treatment of a phase, like menopause, but rather as a life-long therapy for the determent of age-related diseases. The history of estrogen replacement showing the beneficial effects has been documented in over 50 years of medical studies.

With estrogen therapy, it's not *whether* you should be supplementing, but rather what estrogen you should be using. The estrogen chapter will open your eyes to a new concept of "natural" hormone replacement. Compounding pharmacies now have the capability to formulate and dispense bio-identical hormones which exactly match the hormones your body naturally produces. As you read more, you'll understand why it only makes sense to replace something in your body with an exact replica. This book will also respond to many of the hyped-up news reports from the Women's Health Initiative and tell the real story behind the risks and benefits of estrogen replacement.

Progesterone: Another female hormone which works synergistically with estrogen is progesterone. While this hormone is commonly overlooked, it is used to eliminate estrogen's ability to stimulate uterine growth and bleeding. Because of this synergy, progesterone should be viewed as a life-long partner of estrogen. Progesterone further enhances estrogen's beneficial effects on bone, cholesterol, plaque formation, mood disorders and urogenital atrophy. Recent medical research also demonstrates the protective effect of progesterone against breast cancer. Many women who have had hysterectomies are not prescribed progesterone, and therefore lack one very important element of a complete hormone package. Natural progesterone works with estrogen by keeping the prevalent illnesses of aging, like osteoporosis, heart disease and depression at bay. Progesterone has a mild tranquilizing effect and enhances an overall sense of well-being. Studies have shown it to be truly a feel-good hormone.

Testosterone: Although testosterone is the primary male hormone, women also benefit from its supplementation. Levels of testosterone decline in both men and women, and as a result, both gain visceral fat, experience a loss in energy, undergo mood swings, and hopelessly watch as their libido goes out the door. At optimal levels testosterone increases bone density and bone formation, enhances energy and sex drive, decreases body fat, increases muscle strength and size, lowers blood pressure, and positively affects the levels of LDL and HDL. What women may not know is that testosterone keeps their skin soft and supple. Testosterone supplementation is a cost-efficient and emotionally effective tool in curbing the euphemistically termed "midlife crisis". With all of the life benefits testosterone offers, it's a hormone both men and women should not venture into their fifties without.

Thyroid: This metabolic hormone secreted by the thyroid gland regulates temperature, energy, metabolism, and cerebral function. At optimal levels it breaks down fat, resulting in weight loss and lower cholesterol. The thyroid hormone wards off heart disease and memory impairment. Insufficient thyroid levels result in fatigue, slowness in speech and action, depression, and immune dysfunction. Smaller but still perceptible changes also include thinning hair and brittle nails.

Many of these characteristics sound suspiciously like symptoms of getting old. They are, yet they don't have to be. The supplementation of a natural thyroid hormone can alter what is termed "normal" changes seen with aging. Hallmark studies have shown that, even when a patient tests normal for thyroid levels, supplementing a natural source of thyroid can greatly enhance overall well-being. I consider the thyroid one of the most misunderstood and underused hormones in the entire replacement program. The thyroid chapter in this book will go against the grain of traditional medicine: "don't treat a problem if there isn't one." I believe in treating the potential problem so later on there doesn't have to be one to treat. This you will see is the key to preventive medicine.

Natural hormones are pharmaceutical, bio identical (human identical) hormones derived from either plants or synthetically manufactured. In this book, I will refer to "synthetic" hormones as the hormones that are not bio-identical and can have harmful side effects. The words natural and synthetic get confusing. Let's clear up my definitions. When I refer to "synthetic", they are chemically altered hormones, like Provera® (medroxyprogesterone) or Premarin® (conjugated esterified estrogens). These hormones do not match the hormones naturally made by the body. When I refer to "Natural" hormones, they are identical to the hormones found in the body and therefore provide the same physiological effects as our own hormones

A Quick Word of Advice

You may be on a hormone therapy regimen now. If you're a woman, you may already take a form of estrogen and progesterone. Before proceeding further, I recommend you be careful with the type of hormones you take. Many women and men are given the synthetic, chemically altered versions of hormones which are not what our bodies naturally produce. Before you venture further into this book, it is important to understand the difference in semantics and chemical make-up of these two different types of hormones. This is the key to appreciating the controversy and subsequent misunderstandings regarding what hormones are and what they do.

Natural, bio identical hormones are created in a laboratory to exactly match the hormones your body produces. They cannot be patented (no patent means no financial incentive). Synthetic hormones are manufactured to be as close to natural as possible and to mimic the effects of the natural hormones. Unfortunately, even slight altering of the molecular structure could result in unwanted side effects and potential harm. Synthetic hormones can be patented by the pharmaceutical companies and therefore are profitable, in contrast to natural hormones which can not. As physicians, we believe the pharmaceutical industry develops drugs that work. This is certainly not the case with hormones. Synthetic hormones do not work as well and are fraught with side effects and complications. This is exactly what this book is about: contrasting the differences between natural hormones and synthetic hormones for the medical community and lay public to understand.

Throughout this book, my goal is to dispel the myths behind the various types of hormones. I will also attempt to unravel the mysteries of the natural hormones we produce in our youth. These are the exact natural hormones required for supplementation throughout the aging process. Cellular receptor sites are best stimulated by bio identical hormones. This is a simple act of deductive reasoning. Why shouldn't it be considered logical, commonplace medicine? After you read this book I am positive you'll feel the same way.

What You're Up Against

Please be prepared, because adding hormone replacement therapy to your daily routine may prove to be harder than you think. You will probably run into criticism from your family doctor, but not without good reason. For females, the recent Women's Health Initiative Study (WHI) demonstrated an increased risk of breast cancer, heart disease and stroke in women who were treated with the synthetic hormone combination of Premarin® and Provera®. Therefore many physicians do not support the use of female hormones. What they don't understand is that this study does not apply to bio identical hormones, which have different molecular structures, metabolites, and biological effects than the hormones studied in the WHI. Recent and past studies have demonstrated a difference between chemically altered and bio identical hormones. This dissimilarity is not understood by many physicians, journalists and the lay public. We will review the safety, efficacy, and benefits of bio identical hormones based on the medical literature. Large, controlled studies comparing the two groups do not currently exist. Smaller comparison studies are available. We will focus on these comparisons and contrast the health benefit versus detriment. This book is written to educate each patient and each forward thinking physician.

Peer reviewed journals in every specialty of medicine will back me up. I am able to show cardiologists how testosterone, estrogen and thyroid are good for the heart. I am able to show internists that thyroid insufficiencies are not always uncovered by TSH tests, and how thyroid may even help a "healthy" patient. To the doctors looking down their noses at natural hormones, I ask you to read your own journals for the information I extol. The justification is present in our medical journals and literature. The data *for* natural hormones and *against* synthetic hormones is scientific, peer reviewed evidence based in the medical literature.

The idea of perpetuated health throughout life may seem too good to be true. I urge everyone who feels this way to continue reading. This book is not opinion based, nor is it fluff without foundation. Each hormone and its application to longevity medicine are well grounded with clinical backing. This information is on the cusp of breaking into mainstream medicine: not only for the feel-good benefits, but for the tremendous health benefits you will find. I advise you to read on and educate yourself in this exciting field.

Are Hormones Harmful
Or Beneficial?

This chapter should be on the front page of every newspaper educating the world about hormones. The media has twisted and sensationalized information, causing people to believe hormone replacement therapy could be harmful to their health. If you don't act upon what is going to be explained in this chapter, you risk a shorter life. An unhealthy life far more painful and uncomfortable than what you could be living.

Throughout this book, I've presented studies and data to illustrate the benefits of natural hormone replacement. I've demonstrated just how essential they are to good health. Without hormones, our bodies cannot function optimally. Given how immersed I am in the positive life-changing effects of natural hormone replacement, I continue to be amazed when I encounter people who are afraid of hormones, particularly estrogen.

The media has maligned hormone replacement therapy. The real harm occurs when we lose our own hormones. Physicians hesitate to prescribe hormones because the medical journals recommend hormones only to control symptoms and only for the shortest time necessary. They aren't making the most important distinction: these recommendations apply only to synthetic hormones and not to bio- identical hormones. Medical studies demonstrate the harm associated with synthetic hormones and I am in absolute agreement with the medical establishment. Synthetic hormones are dangerous and should not be used. However, the exact opposite is true when it comes to bio identical hormones. The Kaiser organization sent letters to all their female patients recommending that they stop all hormones. This was a severe disservice to these patients. They should have informed their patients about the harmful effects that occur without hormones. They should have advised their patients to stop *synthetic* hormones and switch to the safe, effective, biologically identical hormones.

What happens when hormone replacement is dropped entirely?

- Medical literature demonstrates that after ten years of hormone deprivation, many women will lose their teeth due to loss of mandibular bone support.

- Macular degeneration is an eye disease that causes deterioration of the macula, the part of the eye that processes straight-ahead vision. Macular degeneration is a major cause of blindness. Women who are on estrogen experience 80 percent less macular degeneration and vision loss. This is a protection that women will lose if they stop their hormones.

- Women who have taken estrogen for 15 years or more have a very low incidence of Alzheimer's disease. A recent study demonstrated estrogen's powerful effects in protecting against dementia.

- There is a 50 percent reduction in strokes and heart attacks in women who start estrogen at menopause. Why lose this benefit?

- Estrogen prevents bone loss and osteoporosis. In women 65 years of age or older who suffer hip fractures, 50 percent die within two years. What woman wants this?

- Loss of estrogen produces detrimental changes in the brain, eyes, teeth, bones, heart, blood vessels, cholesterol, skin, and vaginal lining.

Unfortunately, most physicians fail to advise patients of loss of protection against breast cancer, and loss of hair, skin, nails, muscle, strength, energy and well-being.

All menopausal women who are not on estrogen replacement or who have stopped their hormone therapy will face these losses.

Recent studies demonstrate the harmful effects of Provera®. However, recent studies also demonstrate the importance of progesterone in protecting the uterus, breasts, vaginal epithelium, blood vessels and lipids. Maximum breast protection (down-regulation of receptor sites) occurs with high levels of progesterone. Provera® increases breast density, a precursor to cancer. Progesterone decreases breast density, thereby lowering breast cancer risk.

It is the loss of progesterone that increases a woman's risk of cancer. This information is in direct contrast to the way the media and many physicians have interpreted the Women's Health Initiative Study. Women should worry about the loss of progesterone and not the replacement of this incredibly beneficial hormone. Women should fear taking medroxyprogesterone (Provera®).

If hormones were so harmful, physicians would remove every woman's ovaries when she was finished having children. Of course we all know this isn't done! It used to be a common practice to remove ovaries with surgical hysterectomies. The ovaries are now saved whenever possible. When the ovaries are left in place, they continue to produce the health protective hormones until natural menopause.

Recently, we have come to appreciate how important estrogen is for health and well-being. Without ovarian hormones, women face increased incidence of depression, weight gain, accelerated osteoporosis, heart disease and stroke. The longer women go without their hormones, the more they deteriorate. They lose strength, energy, libido, and sense of well-being. A recent study in the medical journal *OB-GYN* demonstrated that there was much less morbidity, mortality, heart disease and osteoporotic fractures in menopausal women who retained their ovaries through menopause compared to those who had their ovaries removed early. Again, ovaries secrete hormones that benefit the body. These hormones should be maintained indefinitely at optimal levels.

The real harm is in losing the hormones that provide so many beneficial effects. The body will experience definite harm when it loses these hormones. The body is also harmed by chemically altered hormones used to replace its own natural hormones. From an evolutionary standpoint it only makes sense that the body does not make hormones harmful to itself.

The medical literature now demonstrates there is no harm from replacing our natural hormones back to optimal levels. The hormones our body naturally produces are always beneficial. Don't allow your body to deteriorate from the lack of hormones. Women need to fear losing estrogen and progesterone and not fear replacing them. I encourage everyone to seize the opportunity to live a healthy and productive life. In spite of the negative media hype, the intent of this book is to dispell the supposition that hormones are harmful and to review the plethora of medical literature in support of maintaining optimal hormone levels in both men and women.

DHEA:
The Age Gauge

People tell me I look better and I know that I feel better. It is like a new lease on life. My doctor can't believe it.

—James, 49

My energy level is unbelievable. I feel as I did when I was thirty.

—Amanda, 56

I'm starting with DHEA (dehydroepiandrosterone) because of its widespread benefit throughout the body. Nicknamed the "Mother of all Hormones" DHEA has the ability to convert into estrogen, testosterone, and progesterone. It has a powerful function apart from being a hormone precursor. This hormone enhances the immune system and modulates   impact on the body, heart and mind. DHEA counters various age-related diseases which can alter the way we age. DHEA is produced by the adrenal glands (glands above the kidneys). Once believed to be a "slacker" hormone, it did not act like any other hormone and appeared to have no direct purpose. DHEA was later seen as the hormone which converted into estrogen, testosterone, or progesterone. The belief was solely that DHEA was a precursor hormone—there to create other hormones, but not serve a purpose of its own. In 1984, Dr. Norman Orentreich proved DHEA declined with age. Scientists then took notice and studies began regarding how DHEA affected age, but more importantly how age affected DHEA.

As an emergency physician, I've seen countless patients over the years in life-threatening situations. I've seen patients in normal situations where aches and pains are discussed quietly in my office. I've saved lives when hearts have stopped and I've saved lives in patients with massive traumas, infections, burns, and gunshot wounds.

All in all, it is rare to receive a thank you in an emergency setting. Yet, when the quality of a patient's life has been radically improved with hormone replacement therapy, the thank you's, hugs, heart-felt cards and long-lasting friendships are just the tip of the rewards. My medical practice has transformed into a life-revival practice. It is extraordinary to watch someone learn to laugh and enjoy life again.

> **Hormone replacement therapy may not be a cure for dying but it makes life longer, exciting, and much more fulfilling. Hormone replacement therapy provides vigor and vitality which would otherwise be lost.**

The message I would like to communicate is that aging doesn't *have* to be the downward spiral you have witnessed in your parents and grandparents. This is the era to look forward to, as you enjoy everything you have worked hard to attain. The transformations are truly remarkable. It is a huge reward to watch old patients renew their lives by transforming complaints into testimonials of revived youth and energy. Hormone replacement therapy may not be a cure for dying, but it makes life more exciting, and much more fulfilling.

We have treated patients on the brink of a physical and emotional meltdown who, with the help of hormone replacement therapy, have experienced renewed energy and sense of well-being, nothing short of a miracle. The stories will make anyone wary because of their too-good-to-be-true nature. Personally, I have experienced real-life examples and am a living proof of what HRT can do. The success stories in our practice are endless. Men approach me with tales of how great they feel on HRT. They typically recount the tiredness and irritability they felt prior to their program. Men express their heart-felt thanks with the revelation they have never felt better. Women are a little different. Their concerns are more focused on aesthetics, metabolism, and health. Nevertheless, women too express their thanks for getting back their lives. Fatigue, loss of libido, changes in hair, skin, and nails become complaints of the past. Our greatest reward is a new patient who explains they want to feel as good as their friend who referred them.

A 52 year-old woman, we'll call her "Susan," came to me already supplementing with progesterone and estrogen but still complaining of general malaise, accompanied with weakness and muscle pain. Her doctor performed every conceivable blood test and dismissed her symptoms as being produced from an overactive imagination, and in turn prescribed her an entourage of 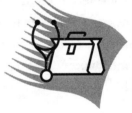 antidepressants. This new diet of mood stabilizers neither enhanced her mood, nor caused any sort of relief from the physical pain she experienced day after day.

Seeing conventional treatments were not offering Susan relief, a friend referred her to me. After reviewing her blood tests, I prescribed her testosterone, DHEA, and thyroid.

With this new regimen, Susan immediately noticed she was no longer fatigued. Her joints and muscles no longer ached. She told me that her children and husband also noticed the difference. Her husband was grateful for her renewed interest in their love life, and her children remarked that it felt like the windows were opened and the air began to flow again within their home. She felt as young and vibrant as she did before menopause.

Stories like these reinforce my desire to encourage and take part in studies focused on the human use of natural hormones.

Every hormone is involved in the complex drama playing out inside our bodies. Individual hormones are not performing their own monologue; rather, all hormones perform with each other, taking cues and signals on when to act or react.

Throughout this book, I focus on each hormone and thoroughly explain the multiple function of that hormone. My hope is everyone interested will understand the benefits of hormone replacement therapy as well as the detrimental effects of suboptimal hormones. Each reader should become educated in the importance of hormone replacement. We will assist our readers in locating a physician who is knowledgeable and passionate about preventive medicine or age-management medicine. With the proper knowledge and motivation, you will hold the key to putting the life back in your years.

Let's Get Technical: DHEA as our Biochemical Clock

Esteemed researcher, Dr. William Regelson of the Medical College of Virginia believes, as do I, DHEA is one of the best, if not the prime, example of a biochemical marker for chronological age. By the time we hit 80, the zona reticularis of the adrenal gland, where DHEA is made, has atrophied, leaving us with 10 to 20 percent of the DHEA levels we once had when we were in our mid-20s.

As with all our vital steroid hormones, such as estrogen, testosterone, and progesterone, DHEA takes its own age-related plunge. This nosedive influences not only the production of the above stated hormones, which of course reflect our gender health, but also the immune system, the 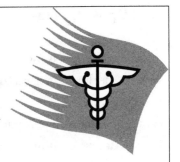 heart, the possibility of cancer and autoimmune disorders, like lupus and rheumatoid arthritis. Along with affecting our sex drive, sense of well being, and physical appearance, DHEA, the once believed slacker hormone, is now thought to be a sort of "age gauge," a hormone that seems to dictate the quality and quantity of years in our lives. Countless studies have rendered DHEA, as not only the most abundant hormone in the human body, but perhaps the most significant hormone for health protection. All major medical journals have published impressive articles on the importance of DHEA in preventing diabetes, heart diseases and cancer. As far as longevity is concerned, this was addressed in the *New England Journal of Medicine* which stated overall morbidity and mortality is directly related to the level of DHEA. High levels of DHEA are associated with increased longevity whereas low DHEA levels are predictive of early mortality. This hormone is very beneficial to health and well-being.

DHEA is one hormone we should never let slip to low levels. It has been shown to inhibit disease, preserve youth and maintain health. There are even such cases as lupus or osteoporosis, where the disease symptoms reverse with the administration of DHEA. I want to begin with the system in the body that is really the culprit behind the advancement of aging—the immune system.

Laid Up With Colds?

DHEA, as well as the efficiency of our immune system, declines at a rapid pace as we reach our thirties. We find ourselves more susceptible to colds and our medicine cabinets become jam-packed with the latest flu remedies. From vitamin combinations to prescription drugs, we're trying our best to beat the odds.

Recently falling hormone levels have been studied as a source for an elderly immune system's sluggish response to foreign invaders. Even more exciting are the studies revealing we can actually rejuvenate an aging immune system and stave off infections with natural hormone replacement therapy. Before I explain how DHEA jumpstarts the immune system, it is necessary to clarify the involved workings of the immune system.

The aging of the immune system is referred to as immunosenescence. Studies are finding that the "normal" age-related immune system decline is not inevitable. DHEA has proven itself time and again to prevent the immune system from becoming idle. With proper supplementation of DHEA, our levels remain youthful, strengthening our immune system for years to come.

DHEA *prevents* deterioration rather than restoring lost organ mass associated with certain aspects of aging. Early supplementation of DHEA forestalls the shrinkage of the thymus gland, allowing you to stop immunosenescence before it starts. There is only one hormone shown through rigorous studies to halt the deterioration of an already aged thymus gland: DHEA. Prevention is the ultimate key to longevity.

Study after study confirms that DHEA is a veritable treatment for the aging immune system. Researchers have found DHEA's regulation of IL-6 may eliminate many age-related conditions. The way we age depends heavily on the health of our immune system. We effectively have the option to inhibit immunosenescence, preventing the aging of our own body.

Stress: The Second Pillar of Age

Stress is such an integral part of our lives. With each passing year, life gets faster and we get more stressed. As these stresses multiply over time, they sometimes leave less of a person in their wake. Most of us internalize stress. We make it our lifelong companion without realizing the slow, methodical destruction on our vital organs and body functions. We seem to believe that stress motivates and facilitates the end result. Reaching ultimate success is not worth the sacrifice of your health.

Being an emergency physician, I am personally aware of the effects of chronic stress. On top of the high-volume activity and apprehension I encounter in the ER, I am also surrounded by contagious illness. I firmly believe my supplementation of hormones, specifically DHEA, has shielded me from many complications associated with the exposure to disease and stress. By participating in a hormone replacement program, I have conquered the normal life expectancy of an emergency room physician and in essence, elongated it. Had I not started hormone replacement therapy at age forty-three, the grueling nights in the ER would turn into more corticosteroids loitering in my blood stream. My T-cells would lack the ability to quickly attack. My immune system would falter; my heart, mind and overall well-being would suffer.

We know DHEA declines with age. We also know our ability to bounce back after a stressful situation deteriorates as corticosteroids continue to climb. It's a compelling argument to say that the dramatic fall of DHEA and the mass production of corticosteroids are closely related.

Let's Get Technical: DHEA's Relationship to Corticosteroids

Dr. Regelson and Dr. Khorram, both leading researchers of hormone replacement therapy, believe that, although DHEA's influence on the immune system does not *directly* impact the center of immune function (the thymus gland), it *indirectly* affects immunity by its relationship with stress hormones, corticosteroids that adversely affect our immune system.

Cortisol and DHEA are inversely related. When cortisol rises, there is a compensating fall in DHEA. When DHEA increases, there is a compensatory fall in cortisol. Even though cortisol is necessary to help the body cope with an occasional stress, too much stress results in too much cortisol. This suppresses DHEA. Loss of DHEA results in shortened longevity due to the increased deteriorations and heart disease. DHEA is required to counter stress and thereby maintain a less detrimental cortisol level.

As DHEA alters the way stress is handled internally, it is

44

reflected in how we handle stress externally. The adrenal gland produces corticosteroids to gear us up for emotional, mental, and physical strenuous activity. It is the stress hormones that offer us the energy for fight or flight. With their help, our blood sugar rises and our heartbeat increases. Our energy level soars, supplying us with the zeal to make the deadline or handle the stress. Unfortunately, our bodies are not as efficient as we would like. Corticosteroids can wreak havoc on the immune system when chronic increased stress results in their constant elevation. Too much cortisol destroys our immune system, causes diabetes, heart disease, weight gain, fatigue, loss of energy, and rapid aging. People fear prednisone and cortisone due to the total body destruction seen in patients who take steroids for asthma or arthritis. Chronic stress can raise cortisol, which results in similar detrimental effects on our immunity, skin, bones, longevity, and quality of life. The longer and greater the stress, the higher the level of cortisol -- the more DHEA becomes suppressed.

Corticosteroids have also been seen to negatively affect the brain. Stress strains the brain's short-term memory. Prior to starting my own hormone replacement program, my short-term memory faltered under a large amount of stress. Taking DHEA, as well as other hormones, helps me handle both physical and mental stress. It appeared as though my brain had undergone a tune-up whether the stress was mental, physical, emotional or surgical related. The body copes by releasing cortisol for short-term coping, which is a built-in survival mechanism. When the body is under stress, it produces DHEA to help balance the effect of cortisol.

DHEA should be considered an important hormone by mainstream medicine for controlling the side effects of excess cortisol. Because it is not a prescription drug, it falls outside the usual prescribing patterns of physicians. The high

DHEA/low corticosteroid ratio is the key to healthy aging. DHEA is an important player in my own hormone replacement regimen because of the hectic life I live. Obviously, I love my life the way it is, and as years pile one on top of the other, I will control the effects of chronic stress. As supported in the medical literature, DHEA makes you feel better, look better and live longer. You have a choice: how will you choose to live, look, and feel in your fifties, sixties, seventies and beyond?

Cancer: The Rooted Disease

The problem with conservative medicine is that many doctors believe if you don't have a disease, why seek treatment? This thought process leaves us sitting ducks, waiting for an illness instead of taking a proactive approach to preserve the precious terrain of our bodies. This concept of medicine has only instigated disease.

With the exception of extreme environmental conditions or predisposed genetic dispositions, it is rare for a child to fall prey to cancer. Children and young adults have hormone levels which amplify the immune system's ability. They search the body like a fine-toothed comb for any disturbance, such as bacteria or cancerous growths. Studies are now beginning to confirm cancer, most times, is an age-related disease. DHEA is a hormone that may be able to thwart certain types of cancer.

We have made leaps and bounds in the science community when it comes to searching for a solution to cancer. Yet, we have not found any definitive cures for this malicious disease. Administering DHEA to laboratory mice has been shown to prevent varied forms of cancer within the breast, lung, colon, liver, skin, and lymphatic tissue. Regelson believed DHEA may show the same benefits in humans. To illustrate his confidence, he tested it on patients. To his delight, he found promising results. DHEA did not cure the cancer, but it borrowed back a few years. To a cancer patient, years are rare jewels.

Like any hormone, self-supplementation is never suggested. DHEA has the ability to convert into testosterone and estrogen. A person with cancer or the potential of cancer should always consult a doctor before purchasing an over-the-counter "cure." Even with these prudent warnings, there is a positive effect seen in the relationship of DHEA and cancer. Amazingly, our own bodies hold the key and provide the hope. As we grow older, a little supplementation of familiar hormones is all it takes to feel healthy again.

A Hearty Hormone

As our hormones take their final bows, dwindling and disappearing from the stage of our body, critical organs and body systems acquiesce to aging's dominance. In short, we begin to die. There are the quintessential outside appearances of age. Graying and thinning hair, wrinkles, age spots, and brittle nails are just some of the visible signs

The odds of developing heart disease skyrockets after we hit the 50-year-old mark. This seems to relate to the decline in our most important hormones. This is DHEA's cue. So how does DHEA sustain a healthy heart and interfere with the natural process of aging? For starters DHEA has the ability to convert to both estradiol and testosterone; this in turn can decrease visceral fat, decreasing the risk of both diabetes and heart disease. Basically DHEA, maintained at youthful levels, keeps bodily systems working in sync.

Several studies have testified to DHEA's powerful ability to curb insulin resistance in women. Diabetes may be a common household name, but there is nothing commonplace about it. DHEA is one of several hormones that may prevent syndrome X and Type 2 diabetes. Obesity plays a large role in the onset of adult diabetes. Sometimes a proper diet and exercise regimen will eliminate these symptoms. I always advocate healthy maintenance of the body and mind, but in some cases this is simply not enough. DHEA has been proven to lower insulin resistance and improve insulin sensitivity. Maintaining optimal levels of DHEA will keep the teeter-totter effect on our side. There is no reason we shouldn't strive to prevent diabetes.

DHEA has also been shown to have some anti-obesity functions. Studies in obese animals have shown that, when supplemented with DHEA, they experience significant weight loss compared to placebo-treated animals. While the studies were done primarily on animals, I have seen the same effects in my patients. This gives hope to those who have tried diet plans and have been unsuccessful in their pursuit for a healthier lifestyle. DHEA is a veritable enemy against age-related fat gain and muscle loss.

Finally, DHEA works as an antioxidant. A recent study in the *Journal of Lipid Research* indicated DHEA had antiatherogenic effects (prevents atherogenesis, the accumulation of lipid containing plaques on the innermost layers of the arteries) through its relation to HDL and LDL lipoproteins.

Age is a formidable enemy of the heart. From insulin resistance to weight gain to cholesterol build-up to stress, the heart is overwhelmed by these enemies. DHEA can be a true protagonist in the story of the heart and an absolute antagonist to the heart's foes. At youthful levels, DHEA keeps insulin in check, is an excellent antioxidant, and buffers the heart against stress.

Adagio for Looking and Feeling Good

At the beginning of this chapter, I told you I loved my job. I will tell you again, there is nothing better than listening to an enthused voice over the telephone telling me they have turned their lives around. They no longer suffer from melancholy and depression and have never felt better.

A 55-year-old banker, Jake, had fallen into the rut of resignation. He felt he needed to retire. He no longer had the drive or passion for job projects. He wanted to go into hiding. His lack of appetite frightened him. He lost his creativity and mental sharpness. He forgot  important dates, deadlines, and projects. His mind and body began to let him down.

Some of his friends had experienced positive results with hormone replacement therapy. Recognizing complacency, they recommended him to my practice. I devised a program consisting of thyroid, testosterone, and DHEA. He began to notice an obvious turnaround. He reported a renewed energy and vigor. He now thrives under pressure again and enjoys beating the odds.

Everyone wants to feel better, yet sometimes people just don't appreciate the health benefits so well-documented in the medical literature.

I've mentioned only in part why our moods suffer. The other part is related to the biology of our endocrine system. The endocrine system is composed of various hormones that in a large part maintain our overall health. Everything related to breathing and thinking depends on the proper function of our hormones. Our hormone levels go through a series of changes over the years, which directly affect the activity of most cells within the body. Whether age is the culprit, or whether our declining hormones incite age, it doesn't really matter. The key issue is: age and decreasing hormones go hand in hand. These are all factors affecting our emotional and intellectual outlook. The decline in mood and thinking ability influences how we age. This is where DHEA supplementation is most beneficial.

Beyond personal patient accounts, there is also a large body of hard, documented proof that DHEA induces a sense of mental and emotional health while promoting stamina. Interestingly enough, the reported increases in mood and energy were not what the tests were conducted to prove. They were added bonuses. In a 1995 University of California School of Medicine study, thirteen men and seventeen women were administered 50 mg of DHEA for six months. Among other benefits, the men and women also reported a "physical and psychological well-being for men (67%) and women (84%)." They attributed this boost of energy and frame of mind to the DHEA which influenced a rise of serum IGF-1 levels and its increased bioavailability to target tissues.

In 1996, a twelve-month study using a DHEA cream on fifteen 60 to 70-year-old women was conducted to determine DHEA's anti-osteoporosis and bone-building benefits. Not only were these hypotheses proven, but 80 percent of women experienced an increase in mood and overall well-being, as well as improved scores for depression and anxiety.

In another more recent 1999 study, M. Bloch et. al. recruited fifteen patients suffering from midlife dysthymia (minor depression). There was a 60 percent positive response during the DHEA phase and only a 20 percent positive response during the placebo phase. There was a general restoration of joy, energy, and motivation. The numbness, sadness and inability to cope with stress that accompanies age were stifled by DHEA's influence.

Many of my new patients complain they no longer enjoy life. They see the years stretch out and their eyes glaze over with a general despondency. They have seen doctors, psychiatrists, herbalists…anyone who may have an answer that works. The usual answer is a prescription mood stabilizer which often creates a neurosis rather than curing one. With a total hormone replacement program, the patient is prescribed natural hormones the body is lacking with the onset of age. DHEA offers great relief from many potential side effects of aging. There are very few potential side effects from its use.

Where to Start

There are only a few things to consider when taking DHEA. High doses are usually well tolerated, although not advised. Few side effects have been reported. Some suffer from moderate acne or hirsutism (increased hair growth in women) . Side effects can be avoided by lowering the dosage.

The fundamental component of hormone replacement therapy is replacing hormones to optimal levels. The key is to replenish all deficient hormones back to a more youthful balance. Which hormones to replenish, how much to replenish and how to adjust the hormone levels to achieve a more youthful level is the art and science of this specialty field of medicine.

DHEA has been through the research wringer for over 40 years. Researchers have not yet uncovered any harmful setbacks. However, there is still apprehension regarding the recommended use. After 40 years of medical studies, there are no studies to show DHEA is harmful. There are 40 years of studies demonstrating the harmful effects of low DHEA levels. As with other hormones, the harmful effects are found in not taking hormones and allowing levels to remain at scientifically proven harmful low levels. These research papers very adequately demonstrate the importance that is often ignored because DHEA is not a drug. Not being a "drug" does not reduce the importance of DHEA.

I have been a part of the experimental process in my own right. DHEA has a long list of proven positive effects. The decline obviously influences many age-related diseases and complications. You now have the proof—not only in stories, but also in studies. You are armed with the knowledge and understanding of DHEA's role in optimal health. Think of the golden years— DHEA can help make these years healthy and happy ones.

In Short...

DHEA's benefits: Boosts the immune system, helps fight stress, is an agent to battle cancer, and helps decrease depression.

DHEA's side effects: Moderate acne, hirsuitism that can be avoided by lowering the dose.

The Bottom Line: When DHEA levels get too low, it can contribute to obesity, diabetes, immune deficiencies, cancer, high blood pressure, and heart disease. Restoring DHEA levels can help reverse all these affects. It may also help improve our learning and give us more energy.

Estrogen:
The Genesis of Hormone
Replacement

*I stopped my hormones after the big scare.
Unfortunately I just couldn't tolerate the hot
flashes and mood swings. I was miserable but
was told it would get better. The joint pains
and soreness just got worse. In just one year I
could feel and see the changes in the skin on
my face. Sex became very uncomfortable. My
best friend referred me to her doctor who put
me on different hormones than before. Soon
thereafter all my symptoms cleared up. Thank
goodness, what a difference. It was a miracle.*
Janis 48

*After my hysterectomy I crashed. Why didn't
someone warn me about this? My OB doctor
ignored my concerns and my family doctor put
me on Premarin®, which helped some. The
antidepressants made me worse and I gained
20 pounds. Finally, my sister forced me to try
her natural hormone program and I can't
believe the difference. I'm back to where I was
before the hysterectomy and the depression is
gone. Estrogen restored my sense of well being.*
Lisa 40

Estrogen—the very hormone that opened the door to
total hormone replacement therapy—has gotten a bad rap
lately. It is not only undeserved, but one which has led many
women to suffer needlessly.

It has become increasingly difficult to get accurate information — information free of sensationalism — into the minds of women and their doctors. In the spring of 2003, the Women's Health Initiative study demonstrated increased risks of heart attacks, strokes, breast cancer and dementia. Across the nation, women quit their hormones while doctors shrugged their shoulders and offered no alternatives. They didn't do what would have most benefited their patients: introduce the concept of bio identical hormones, the concept that I will explore in this chapter.

It was the difficulties of menopause that first brought hormone replacement into the limelight. For more than forty years, doctors prescribed estrogen to women suffering from menopausal symptoms such as hot flashes, vaginal dryness, problems with concentration and anxiety, and insomnia. Estrogen replacement therapy proved to be so effective, some women continued taking the hormone even after menopause. These women felt better and looked better. They were living longer, happier and healthier lives. Aside from the cosmetic benefits—stronger hair, smoother skin, and improved muscle tone—estrogen also decreased their risk of osteoporosis, heart disease, and colon cancer. It was the unanticipated benefits like these that led doctors to take a closer look at the role hormones play in health and aging.

Why should we use estrogen? For starters it protects against or reduces the effects of:
- Heart disease
- Stroke
- High cholesterol
- Alzheimer's Disease

- Memory loss
- Menopausal symptoms
- Osteoporosis
- Urinary tract atrophy
- Skin atrophy
- Depression and mood swings

For decades, women and their doctors treated menopause as a period in life considered to be a natural transition into old age. Instead, it is a condition that can easily be transformed into a rite of passage into a dynamic second adulthood. Women are now living 30 to 40 years beyond menopause. This time in their life needs critical attention and research. For women to avoid a dramatic slide during and after menopause, they must find the resources to enhance the years to come. Estrogen and progesterone appear to be their answer.. They are not only effective, but have been shown to *exceed* expectations, allowing women to feel energized once again.

Estrogen is an essential hormone that not only confronts the uncomfortable symptoms of menopause, but also helps maintain a healthy and youthful environment within the body. Estrogen replacement therapy is a safe and effective treatment against the numerous complications of aging. Natural estrogen replacement is a genuine ally, bolstering bone health, preventing heart disease, and protecting against Alzheimer's disease. It's a woman's safeguard from the signs, symptoms and diseases which accompany age.

In this chapter, my goal is to increase your awareness of the insurmountable proof of natural estrogen's benefits to the female body. The benefits far outweigh the risks. Your main risk is not optimally replacing estrogen. The risks described in the WHI trial were based on the use of the synthetic estrogen. These risks have never been demonstrated with the use of bio identical estrogen. Starting with the benefits and moving forward to the risk, the major differences between natural and synthetic forms of estrogen and progesterone will become clear.

Women are living longer lives and deserve to live free of bone loss, heart complications, and Alzheimer's disease. I stand by the powerful benefits natural estrogen provides for the female body. When you're through reading this chapter, I hope you will understand how natural hormones support the body beyond middle age. As we address the Women's Health Initiative and the truth of those findings, it is important to clear up the confusion between synthetic and natural estrogen. It's not just a matter of semantics but a matter of optimal health.

As a patient or a physician, please use this book as your resource. It is written to help unravel the hype that came out of skewed studies. Educate yourself so you can participate in estrogen replacement free of fear. Enjoy a healthier and happier life.

Since the WHI Trial was published, several other studies have demonstrated that estrogen, whether synthetic or natural, does not cause strokes or heart disease when started soon after menopause. Where estrogen was used by itself, it protected against both heart disease and strokes.

If estrogen were harmful we would remove every woman's ovaries at age 30. We not only don't do this, but make every effort to

> **Don't fear estrogen.**
> **Fear the loss of estrogen.**

leave ovaries in place when performing hysterectomies. Why? Because women experience negative symptoms and develop heart disease and bone loss after the removal of ovaries. Studies now show estrogen and other hormones are so beneficial that ovarian function should be preserved for as long as possible. When the ovaries finally stop working, we optimize levels using natural hormone replacement. Don't fear estrogen. Fear the loss of estrogen.

The Women's Health Initiative

The publication of the Women's Health Initiative findings created a panic. Approximately 50 percent of hormone users discontinued their therapy. This was often without consulting their doctors, and without a clear understanding of what the Women's Health Initiative was reporting. Many doctors failed to understand the study methodology and encouraged their patients to discontinue hormone treatment. As women again began suffering from hot flashes, vaginal dryness, mood swings and depression, they returned to risky synthetic hormones for relief. Their doctors prescribed substances known to be harmful when there was a safe, natural alternative.

The unfortunate result of the hype and panic following the WHI publication is this: women are missing out on the incredible benefits of estrogen. This choice is based on fear and perceived risks. Fear is a natural response. However, the risks are far more minimal than publicized. The increased risk of breast cancer was less than one person per thousand. Nevertheless, there was a slight risk. This risk was only based on Premarin® and Provera® together. The WHI demonstrated no increased risk of breast cancer when taking estrogen by itself.

The Women's Health Initiative was a study that focused on synthetic estrogen (Premarin®) and progestin (Provera®). Provera® is Progestin. Progestin is NOT Progesterone. There were different arms of the study using different drug combinations. The arm of the study using Premarin® and Provera® (PremPro®) demonstrated an increased risk of breast cancer which was detected in the early stages of the study. This risk is attributed to the Provera® portion of the regimen and not the estrogen. This is not the first time progestins have been implicated in increasing risks in women. A *Journal of the American Medical Association* (JAMA) article also notes that Premarin® contains ten estrogens not found in the human body. Three recent studies have demonstrated an eight-fold increased risk of cancer when Provera® was added to estrogen. There is no doubt: Provera® increases the risk of breast cancer. Even though the WHI trial, the most powerful study to date, demonstrated a decreased risk of breast cancer with estrogen replacement only, estrogen replacement always carries the blame.

The only harm demonstrated in the estrogen-only arm was a slightly increased risk of stroke. This was only seen in older women (65 and over) who started HRT after age 65. This was not seen in younger women (under 60) nor in any women who started estrogen within 5 years of menopause. Multiple other studies confirm a decreased risk of heart attacks, heart disease, and strokes in younger women who took estrogen alone.

Multiple studies confirm Premarin® increases clotting in arteries and veins of the heart, legs and lungs. A recent study in JAMA confirmed the same results. Yet, this study also found estradiol (natural estrogen) did not increase risk of clotting in any artery or vein. The increase in clotting seen with Premarin® was demonstrated to be associated with the horse estrogen, equilin.

Unfortunately, the media has misrepresented the facts of this study by targeting all hormone therapy. This is wrong! Again, the culprits are synthetic progestin (Provera®) and horse estrogen (Premarin®). Natural estrogen and natural progesterone are not the culprits. There are numerous studies showing the long-term benefits of hormone therapy. Women need to make sure that they are receiving natural bio identical hormones in the exact dosages. Proper balance is essential for a hormone replacement program.

It is important to begin hormone replacement as soon as your hormones begin to decline. This will prevent a lapse in their protective benefits. Researchers who conducted a study published in the *Journal of General Internal Medicine* noted the mean age of women in the Women's Health Initiative was 63 years old. The average age was 67. Many of these women over 60 did not start hormone replacement at the onset of menopause. In their study, they found that hormone replacement reduced mortality in participants who were under 60 years of age. They also found no change in mortality with women who were over 60 years. In 2003, there were several reports that the findings of the Women's Health Initiative may not apply to younger postmenopausal women on hormone replacement. Women less then 60 demonstrated a decreased risk of heart attack and stroke while on estrogen.

Not Just a Matter of Semantics

There is some confusion over definitions. By now you've heard the adjectives "natural" or "synthetic," and wonder about their true meaning. I hope to clear up any misinterpretation you may have. Many doctors incorrectly assume all hormones are the same. Other doctors criticize natural hormones as worthless and claim synthetic hormones are best. Both of these assumptions are incorrect.

When I use the phrase "natural estrogen replacement" or "natural progesterone replacement," or simply combine the two into the phrase "natural hormone replacement," I am talking about bio identical hormones. Bio identical hormones match the chemical make-up of the hormones your body naturally produces. The term "natural" has been used loosely. Some patients as well as doctors believe "natural" refers to products derived from plants and sold in health food stores. Many fruits, vegetables, grains, nuts, herbs, and spices produce substances called phytoestrogens. These products have minor estrogenic capabilities. Some companies purport these "natural" products can eliminate menopausal symptoms. The truth is even the strongest phytoestrogens have about one to two percent of the potency of human estrogens. They are quite different from natural hormones, prescribed by a physican and compounded in a pharmacy. Natural Hormones are identical to the hormones produced by our body.

The most common synthetic hormones are conjugated estrogens derived from pregnant mares' urine. This is marketed under the brand name Premarin® and is widely used by women and clinics across the United States. These are equine hormones which are very different from human hormones. Medical studies have demonstrated that they function differently than our own hormones. They cause side effects and problems not seen from our own hormones. These horse estrogens may be healthy to horses but they are certainly detrimental to the human body. There is nothing natural about supplementing a female human with female horse hormones or any other synthetic hormone. There are several other reasons synthetic estrogen is not the ideal choice for the female body.

Bio identical hormones are indistinguishable from human hormones as they are molecularly identical. They are produced from a natural plant source, but it is their identical chemical structure that makes them natural. The body recognizes such hormones as identical to what it naturally produces. And, I ask you, what is more natural than something precisely formulated to fit your body?

Why do doctors and women continue to use synthetic alternatives? The answer is a combination of ignorance and price. Natural supplements such as vitamins and bio identical hormones are protected by federal regulation and cannot be patented. Pharmaceutical companies can't profit so they do not have an interest. Pharmaceutical companies specialize in patentable drugs which are exclusive and profitable. Most continuing physician education is from drug companies promoting their products. With limited advertising for bio identical hormones, few doctors are knowledgeable about them. Bio identical hormones are not marketed under specific brand names. A doctor must be proficient in natural hormone replacement to ensure that a patient is prescribed the proper dosage for adequate blood serum levels. Natural hormones are worthless if a patient does not absorb each hormone properly, or if they are not prescribed in adequate amounts.

When synthetic hormones were first developed, they were well-received. They provided benefits by controlling the miserable symptoms of menopause. The long-term results have now shown synthetic hormones elicit harmful effects. There are women who cannot tolerate synthetic hormones. They often suffer side effects such as breast pain, bloating, bleeding, breakouts, and mood swings.

Synthetic hormones are not a perfect match in the body. Synthetic hormones produce abnormal metabolites that can cause side effects and increase the risk of cancer. A natural hormone is a perfect fit in the body—it is a biologically identical hormone the body recognizes as its own.

Estrogen: The What's, How's, and Why's

Estrogen is primarily a female hormone produced in the ovaries and adrenal glands. Estrogen supplementation increases a woman's likelihood for a long life by balancing HDL and LDL levels, maintaining calcium in the bone, preserving the blood vessels' youthful elasticity and keeping the arteries free and clean of the deadly plaque that causes heart disease.

Let's Get Technical: Estrogen

The female body produces three types of estrogen: estrone, estradiol, and estriol. Estradiol is the strongest of all the estrogens and the most abundant during the reproductive years. After menopause, estrone takes center stage as the predominant estrogen.

Estriol is the metabolic byproduct of the two with the weakest estrogenic effect. These three estrogens, through direction of the hypothalamus, work in unison throughout a woman's life to protect her in her adolescent years, her reproductive years, and after menopause by way of 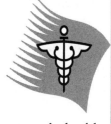 supplementation. Estradiol is most vital to women's health, while estriol and estrone have more minor roles.

Menopause is not the only hormone-buster women need to worry about. Many women undergo full or partial hysterectomies. A partial hysterectomy will remove the uterus and preserve all or part of the ovaries. A full hysterectomy will remove the uterus and ovaries. This will bring on menopause surgically rather than naturally. A woman will immediately begin to suffer menopausal symptoms. To avoid a crash from the sudden cessation of their own hormones, women who have undergone a full hysterectomy should immediately supplement estrogen, progesterone, and testosterone.

Most women who have undergone a hysterectomy notice a dramatic change. Coupled with the trauma of radical surgery, this can be devastating. The quote by "Lisa" at the beginning of this chapter is how women feel after a full hysterectomy. Too many women are placed on antidepressants to mask the effects, when in fact a natural hormone replacement program should be prescribed. Without these vital, health-sustaining hormones, women who have experienced full hysterectomies are in just as much danger as women who have gone through natural menopause. Both groups are susceptible to heart disease, osteoporosis and age related dementia. A severe decline in the quality of their life is another frequent complaint. Women who undergo a partial hysterectomy and retain their ovaries have hormone production until traditional menopause takes place. At that time, they too will need hormone replacement.

With or without ovaries, it is crucial for women to balance their hormones and maintain optimal levels. Regardless of how or when you experience menopause, the years after depend on the supplemental benefits of natural estrogen, progesterone, and testosterone.

The Menopause Cure-all

As a woman's estrogen levels begin to decrease, usually during her mid- to late- forties, she may start to experience discomfort. Many women complain of hot flashes, vaginal dryness, insomnia, poor concentration, weight gain and changes in skin and hair texture. Some of these troublesome symptoms disappear late into menopause. However, at this point, there is an increased risk of cardiovascular disease, stroke, osteoporosis, and Alzheimer's. All of these are severe problems most newly menopausal women are unaware of until it's too late.

Seventy-five percent of all peri-menopausal, menopausal, and late menopausal women suffer from hot flashes. A hot flash is a sudden shock of warmth followed by perspiration and sometimes heart palpitations. For some women, these sudden jolts of heat are minor, but for others they can be absolutely debilitating. We're not exactly sure of the mechanism behind this surge of heat, but we are positive it is directly linked to the sudden shortage of estrogen. Women report that it strikes without warning and is gone before they know it. Although they may be quick, they can be disorienting and embarrassing.

This is the main reason estrogen replacement therapy got underway. It would allow women to ride out menopause without experiencing the bothersome symptoms. Estrogen supplementation eliminates these flare-ups in a matter of days, restoring a woman's self-confidence and composure in everyday situations. Unfortunately, too many women used estrogen as a temporary fix for menopause, rather than a long-term means to increase their quality of life. The advantages of this extended health benefit far outreaches the convenient quick-fix estrogen offers during early menopause.

Along with hot flashes and night sweats, menstrual irregularities start to occur. For most women their period is a sign of health, but during perimenopause the monthly cycle goes awry. Periods can range 25 to 60 days apart. Some periods are light, others are heavy. Don't let this alarm you. Your body is adjusting to the sudden lack of hormones. This stage is termed perimenopause. Abnormal or irregular menstruation during this phase is considered normal.

Many women also complain of mood swings, and this symptom seems to receive more press than any other trait of the menopausal process. Since estrogen interacts with beta-endorphins in the brain (the neuropeptides that curtail pain while enhancing a sense of well-being), the amount of it in the body influences how a woman will view and react to her surroundings. Good moods and balanced emotions in the beginning of the menstrual cycle are attributed to estrogen's high levels. Loss of estrogen causes unprovoked episodes of crying even at a minor irritation.

As a woman gets older and estrogen levels begin to decline, it's no surprise her mood deteriorates. With the erratic aspect of a woman's hormones during perimenopause, and the intersection of these crazed hormones with the ongoing process of life, some women become overwhelmed and depressed.

I remember, in particular, a woman sitting in my office with a balled-up tissue in one hand and a bottle of prescription mood-stabilizers in the other. I'll call her Rebecca. She had been put on Prozac to curtail her "mood disorder" when she was forty-five. At age forty-six she was sitting in my office at the urging of a co-worker with tears streaming down her face.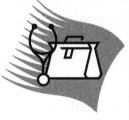

Rebecca believed she was doomed, and her husband believed he had married Dr. Jeckyl and Mr. Hyde. After having her blood drawn and tested, I was able to assure Rebecca she did not have a split personality, she was simply lacking the proper levels of the hormone essential for her emotional health.

After three weeks on a combination of estriol, estradiol and progesterone she visited me without her Kleenex and gone was the hopelessness that seemed to enshroud her less than a month before. She mentioned that she felt as if a heavy wool blanket had been removed from her shoulders, like she could breathe again.

Estrogen has proven itself to be a veritable solution to the menopausal blues. In a double-blind, placebo-controlled study, women supplemented with estrogen and progesterone demonstrated an increase of well-being via their results on the

Profile of Adaptation to Life test and a decrease in depression measured via their results on the Beck Depression Inventory.

Other symptoms, such as vaginal dryness and urinary infections, can also be side-stepped with estrogen supplementation. Since the entire genitourinary tract is lined with estrogen receptors, an estrogen deficiency creates negative changes in the vagina's environment. The mucosa does not as readily lubricate the vagina when sexually aroused, compromising the prospect of intimacy. It is just too painful, and therefore uninviting. I've had many patients tell me they felt guilty because they no longer desired sex, and with the mood swings they felt they were on totally different planets than their husbands. The husbands remained intimate, yet the women wanted nothing of the sort.

Not only does the mucosa stop functioning correctly, but the vaginal entrance becomes smaller and thinner. This process makes sexual intercourse not only painful but impossible for many women. This is called "vaginal atrophy," where the walls become insubstantial and the actual vagina becomes shorter and narrower. A woman at thirty may have fifty to sixty vaginal layers, while a woman of eighty years of age may only have eight. As the skin thins, the cells that maintained the delicate acidic balance become more alkaline, putting the vagina at risk for bacteria to cause infection. The thinning also exposes the vagina to chafing, leaving a woman prone to develop urinary and vaginal infections. Estrogen limits this effect by restoring vaginal tone and elasticity. It increases blood flow and enhances the vagina's lubricating ability. Sex is a natural human hunger, and menopause should not be the final curtain on such an essential and enjoyable aspect of a woman's life.

Another benefit to estrogen therapy is the positive influence it has on the skin. We have heard the phrases "aging gracefully", or "she ages well." The cardinal physical signs of aging reside in the skin, which becomes dry, thin, and wrinkled – changes which are emotionally unsettling for some women. This especially happens to women after menopause. For years, the dermatology literature has demonstrated estrogen's protective benefits on skin by prevention of the severe atrophy and thinning commonly seen after menopause. The paper-thin skin found on the arms of all older women not on hormones is due to loss of collagen when there is no estrogen or testosterone to maintain it.

How estrogen therapy helps women maintain thicker, healthier skin is quite simple. Estrogen stimulates the production of hyaluronic acid on collagen which helps hold water and moisture in the inner layer of skin. This in turn supports the outer layer of skin allowing more elasticity while maintaining the overall firmness. This is truly encouraging news to every disheartened woman who notices her skin beginning to sag. Women no longer have to spend their life's savings on creams, sprays and cosmetic treatments. Estrogen naturally tightens and firms sagging skin.

Natural estrogen inhibits the common symptoms a large number of women feel as they pass through the menopausal years. Forty years of successful therapy have proven that hot flashes, insomnia, mood swings, vaginal dryness, and skin atrophy can be eliminated through estrogen supplementation.

What estrogen does for the body before and during menopause is truly amazing. My primary concern as a doctor - and your uppermost interest as a maturing woman - is the years after menopause, where aging without estrogen can truly undermine your health. By breaking aging's chain of events through estrogen supplementation, you can avoid such illnesses as osteoporosis, heart disease, and Alzheimer's. Let's see how.

Osteoporosis: A Breakthrough for Healthy Bones

Uncomfortable symptoms are only the beginning when it comes to menopause. This is not the only reason women must include estrogen in their personal hormone regimen. Another reason is the rapid loss of bone mass after menopause which has been directly linked to declining levels of estrogen. Science has now uncovered estradiol's important role in bone formation and has found receptor sites for estrogen in the female's skeletal structure. Estrogen is also important to the body's ability to utilize calcium, an essential ingredient for healthy bones. In all of these ways, estrogen has demonstrated a clear-cut benefit for preventing and treating osteoporosis.

Let's Get Technical: What our Bones Do

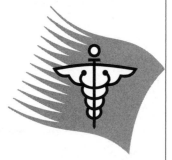

Bone is dynamic tissue and each year 10 percent of it turns over, meaning new bone replaces the old. Women hit their peak bone mass about the age of thirty-five. From then on, although the bones still rebuild, women lose more bone than they're able to make. As women age, their bodies process less new bone for old bone. The inner part of the bone, the trabecular bone, gets thinner while the outer bone, the cortical bone, retains its original shape. A hollowing occurs, and bones become brittle.

In human bodies, cells called osteoclasts and osteoblasts continually tear down and rebuild bones. (Osteoclasts tear down old bone while osteoblasts build new.) As we age, the osteoclasts start outworking the bone-building osteoblasts, and we begin losing bone mass. For women, however, these losses can double or even quadruple, from about 1 percent per year to 2-4 percent during the decade following menopause. The result is osteoporosis, or "porous bones."

Osteoporosis is more or less a silent disease that is usually undetected until after the damage has been done. About 24 million Americans suffer from osteoporosis, and 80 percent of those are women, especially older women. Osteoporosis cripples a woman's ability to live a healthy and active lifestyle. In some cases, complications arise after injuries such as hip fractures. Unfortunately, hip fractures kill a substantial number of osteoporosis sufferers in the United States each year.

There are certain bones that seem more easily lured into osteoporatic loss. The hip and wrist become fragile. Osteoporosis causes the vertebral bone, the bone in your back, to collapse in, resulting in a hunching over, or what is referred to as "dowager's hump." The scary part of this is that it usually takes four to five crushed vertebrae for a person to become aware of this debilitating and advanced disease.

The good news is that natural estrogen eliminates a woman's risk of osteoporosis. Estrogen fine-tunes the process of bone remodeling by stimulating the release of calcitonin and vitamin D as well as enabling calcium to be deposited back into bone.

Let's Get Technical: Calcitonin

Calcitonin, from the thyroid gland, inhibits osteoclasts, which slows down remodeling, maintaining adequate bone mass. Vitamin D helps the body absorb calcium from food and stimulates the kidneys to reabsorb calcium from the urine.

This is one of the unexpected benefits doctors discovered in women who were taking estrogen for menopausal symptoms. Results of the Postmenopausal Estrogen/Progestin Interventions Trials (PEPI), found that women taking estrogen gained bone density, and most had no bone loss at the spine or hip.

Osteoporosis can be a disabling disease. Women diagnosed with osteoporosis find themselves concerned about their safety during activities they once considered normal. As bones become too brittle, stepping off a curb or twisting in the most common way can cause a hip-fracture. Osteoporosis is an entirely preventable disease. Estrogen is truly a boon for the bone. Not only does it have its own receptor sites within the bone, estrogen oversees and puts into action the body's skeletal blueprint, a never-ending construction project. Estrogen allows a woman to climb stairs, open a jar of pickles, or pick up her grandbaby without a second thought or trepidation of fracturing her hip or spine.

Since women are at a higher risk for osteoporosis than men they need to take the proper precautions and include estrogen in their health-maintenance regimen. It is first-line therapy that should be started in early menopause and continued throughout a woman's lifetime. Estrogen not only defines the curves on a younger woman's body, it also defines a mature woman by allowing her to stand taller and stronger as she ages and begins the adventure into the second half of her life.

Harnessing Heart Disease

Another pleasant surprise doctors discovered is that women taking estrogen can cut their risk of heart disease by as much as 50 percent. Estrogen's heart-healthy attributes were discovered over forty years ago. At that time, doctors observed that women who had their ovaries removed became as susceptible to heart disease as men. Heart disease is only a minor threat to younger women. However, as they pass into menopause—and estrogen levels dip—heart disease becomes the number one killer of both men and women. Heart disease is no longer a male-dominated disease. Currently, almost half of all women die of heart disease in America. It is the most formidable enemy a middle-aged woman will face. Fortunately, it can be fought by replacing estrogen to optimal levels which were protective in her pre-menopause years.

Estrogen supplementation can also increase insulin sensitivity, which bars the door against adult onset diabetes. This is good news for women as diabetes actually doubles a woman's chance of developing heart disease. How does this work? When insulin resistance occurs, the body makes up for it by creating more insulin. This overproduction can cause increased plaque formation in the blood vessels thereby increasing the risk of heart disease and stroke. Mounting evidence shows estrogen decreases the incidence of both diabetes and heart disease. The Nurses Health Study reported, among other health advantages, that women who took estrogen had a twenty percent decrease in the incidence of diabetes.

Estrogen works in a number of ways to help reduce the risk of heart disease. Estrogen can help lower LDL (low density lipoprotein) "bad cholesterol," while raising HDL, (high density lipoprotein), the "good cholesterol." Estrogen may also help protect the heart and arteries through its effect as a free radical scavenger. Some doctors and scientists believe that if we were able to effectively master free radical damage, we could add years to a human's life. Like vitamins E and C, estrogen acts as a powerful antioxidant and limits the oxidative damage to the arteries that causes plaque.

What do these studies show us? They demonstrate that estrogen can be a key ingredient to a healthy heart. Many women, who avoid hormone replacement because they are afraid of the risks, are on a headlong journey toward heart complications.

> **Many women who avoid hormone replacement because they are afraid of its risks are on a headlong journey toward heart complications.**

All of these life-saving aspects of estrogen are only realized so long as a woman continues to take estrogen and maintains optimal blood levels of the hormone. In just months after a woman stops her estrogen replacement program, the risks will again escalate. With the statistics of heart disease mortality as they are and the proof-positive results of estrogen therapy, it is startling that so many women lack vital knowledge about this life-saving hormone. Too many women are not reaping the benefits of natural hormone therapy. Your heart has been shielded by estrogen for the years before menopause. As shown in the studies above, without estrogen to fine-tune the complex workings of the heart, vessels harden (atherosclerosis), plaque forms, and heart disease becomes the dominant force which will ultimately kill 60 percent of women.

Estrogen is perhaps the most vital part in maintaining a woman's healthy heart. In matters of the heart, estrogen replacement therapy has illustrated an impressive track record—so impressive both the American Heart Association and the American College of Cardiology have issued guidelines recommending physicians take into account the use of estrogen replacement therapy as a means to prevent or treat cardiovascular disease. The result of the WHI trial demonstrated increased risk of heart disease and stroke when estrogen and progestins were used in older women. This does not apply to women taking bio identical hormones or to women who start hormone supplementation at menopause. The results of the WHI cannot be extrapolated to include younger women on other hormones. Forty years of studies document estrogen's beneficial effect at reducing heart disease and strokes. Since the WHI trials, all other studies demonstrate reduced risk of stroke and heart attack.

Brain Food

As research continues into the role hormones play in our bodies and the potential benefits of hormone replacement, scientists are confirming that when it comes to hormones, what's good for the body is good for the brain. Although estrogen was never meant to be a preventative therapy or treatment for dementia, what studies have found is nothing short of exciting. Women on estrogen therapy often report an improvement in mood and feeling of well-being. They also sense an increase in their memory. Science is showing this stems from more than just the relief that comes with treating the symptoms of menopause. Multiple medical studies have demonstrated improved cognition and memory in women taking estrogen.

It's interesting that some women, who have never had a problem with depression, feel a sudden shift with the onset of menopause. This is not surprising since estrogen is the body's own natural mood stabilizer. The pharmaceutical industry has formulated antidepressants, like Prozac and Zoloft, which do what optimal levels of estrogen have done all along—inhibit the serotonin-metabolizing enzyme and monoamine oxidase (MAO), while allowing the neurotransmitter serotonin to travel freely and elevate mood. Estrogen, indeed, works on mood health by increasing serotonin levels to prevent and treat depression.

Many of my patients have attested to a renewed optimistic outlook while on estrogen therapy. Numerous studies have validated their claims.

Countless studies have demonstrated estrogen's positive effects on memory and learning, as well as other mental processes. Since women make up 72 percent of the population over the age of eighty-five, researchers are now taking a hard look at how estrogen may also reduce the risk of Alzheimer's disease. There are a few distinctive features of Alzheimer's disease. Although it is normal for neurons to gradually decrease with age, in an Alzheimer's victim the rate of loss is significantly greater especially in regions of the brain associated with memory and learning. Alzheimer's disease is due to the deposition of a beta-amyloid protein in neurons causing neurofibrillary tangling and destruction of neurons. Estrogen has overwhelmingly demonstrated its power to prevent this damage and prevent Alzheimer's disease.

Many other studies show similar effects on mental function and cognition in women who do not have Alzheimer's. Thus, estrogen use protects against the pathology that causes Alzheimer's. It also protects the brain from the routine memory loss that is typically encountered by most of us through the aging process.

Whatever the case, the fact that estrogen can prevent Alzheimer's is great news for every woman. Research into Alzheimer's and estrogen is ongoing and so far estrogen has been the only therapy known which dramatically protects against Alzheimer's. Study after study has shown proof-positive results that the supplementation of estrogen prevents Alzheimer's disease. As a doctor of preventive medicine, it is not enough to just extend the years of a patient's life. My goal is to also extend the quality of their life.

The Estrogen Scare: Breast and Ovarian Cancer

Estrogen has picked up some bad press—especially after the flawed reporting of the Women's Health Initiative. Some doctors and scientists still speculate that estrogen causes breast cancer. These claims are showing up in headlines and news stories across the nation.

The Rouzier camp focuses on a different thought process altogether. What many news articles seem to omit is the fact that the estrogen-only arm of the study showed a decreased incidence of breast cancer. It was only the combination of Premarin® and Provera® that showed an increase in cancer. This initiative proved estrogen alone does not cause cancer -- it is the addition of Provera® that is dangerous. Nonetheless, the world still believes estrogen is the culprit. In my practice, I do not personally recommend Premarin® or Provera® but am obligated to explain the actual risk of breast cancer when one chooses to take these synthetic hormones. The increased risk of breast cancer is very small, less than one per thousand. This means out of 1000 women who took Premarin® and Provera®, only one would be expected to develop cancer and the remaining 999 would not. Throughout the medical community, this is not explained very well.

The risk of getting breast cancer is slim, but that hardly makes for an exciting news flash. Well, here is a news flash — the leading cause of death in women is heart disease and stroke (60 percent). Heart disease far surpasses the risk of breast cancer. Women are terrified of breast cancer but remain unaware heart disease is the leading cause of death.

The WHI trials demonstrated estrogen alone did not increase the risk of cancer or heart disease. The plain-as-day fact that estrogen protects the heart from disease cannot be disputed. Estrogen saves lives. Sadly, the truth is stained by the supposed threat of breast cancer and heart disease. Women see the word cancer and everything else fades to a blur. Let's put things back into perspective and sharpen your focus—present-day data confirms that the paranoia over breast cancer is just that—paranoia. Natural estrogen does not cause breast cancer.

In the previous segments of this chapter, I illustrated through clinical data the life-saving benefits a woman can reap from estrogen replacement. I have shown you what estrogen can do; now I would like to talk about what estrogen does not do. I also want to help women understand that taking estrogen after breast cancer does not add fuel to the fire. In many cases, estrogen has been shown to actually increase a breast cancer victim's chance of survival. Then why the big scare—and where did doctors come up with the idea that estrogen causes breast cancer? Most studies have not made a distinction as to whether Premarin® or Premarin® in combination with Provera® was used. Therefore most studies are combined studies and would be expected to show an increase in breast cancer. Thus there are some studies demonstrating a risk of cancer and some studies showing no risk of cancer. The WHI study demonstrated an increased risk with Premarin® and Provera®, whereas there was a decreased risk using estrogen alone!

Twenty years ago, in 1987, researchers of the Cancer and Steroid Hormone Study observed women on estrogen therapy for twenty years or longer. They found no increased incidence of breast cancer, not even in women who had a positive family history of breast cancer. "Overall, the risk of breast cancer did not appear to increase appreciably with increasing HRT duration or latency, even for durations and latencies of 20 years or longer."

Another more recent study featured in the American Journal of Preventive Medicine showed an analysis from the NHANES (First National Health and Nutrition Examination Survey) I Epidemiology Follow-up Study that concluded there was no increased risk for breast cancer in women who used HRT. They found no statistically significant association between HRT and the development of breast cancer in the

5,761 women who participated in the study from 1971 to 1992.

It is very interesting that women who take oral contraceptives containing two to four times higher doses of estrogen and progestin than that found in hormone replacement therapy have no significant increase in breast cancer. In a 1985 issue of *Lancet*, a study concluded women under the age of 45 did not experience an aggregate risk of breast cancer when taking a form of oral contraceptive.

Many women, who have or have had breast cancer, are curious about whether they can partake in estrogen's many life-saving benefits. Many of their doctors will say no. Once a woman has had breast cancer, it is common practice to avoid hormone replacement.

> **Many studies are now showing that women who have survived breast cancer need not be deprived of estrogen's life-saving assistance.**

These women not only have suffered the trauma of breast cancer, but now must face a life without the heart healthy, bone building and mood-enhancing benefits of estrogen. Many studies are now showing women who have survived breast cancer need not be deprived of estrogen's life-saving assistance. Several women who used hormone replacement or an oral contraceptive at the time of their breast cancer diagnosis showed improved survival rates over women who did not. There are more than 60 studies demonstrating estrogen is safe if given 5 years after breast cancer treatment. In all of these studies, there were no increased cancer recurrences. In fact there were decreased recurrences as well as less heart disease and increased survival.

What is proven? Estrogen maintains heart health, builds bone, perhaps (as far as initial studies are concerned) aids in cognition and emotional ailments common in the elderly and eliminates the menopausal blues. Too many women are missing out on these life-altering benefits. Physicians and patients remain confused over the cancer issue which stems from misunderstanding the combination of Premarin® and Provera®. Unfortunately, the focus is on the fear of breast cancer and not on the harmful results from loss of estrogen.

Estrogen has received a bad rap when it comes to the subject of cancer. Have you heard recently that estrogen helps deter colon cancer? Colon cancer is more common in women than in men and is one of the leading causes of cancer incidence and deaths in women. Many studies have focused on estrogen's effect on colorectal cancer. These studies have shown that with continued use, estrogen protects against the incidence of colon cancer. It's unknown exactly how estrogen is protective. Some think it might be that estrogen affects bile acid metabolism or promotes tumor suppressor activity. Colon cancer is far more prevalent in women than breast cancer. Women often do not realize that estrogen can provide protection against colon cancer.

So, why do we only get the negative side of the story? It beats me. Estrogen is such a dynamic and essential hormone offering both short- and long-term benefits. It's amazing that many women perceive only the possible risks and never recognize the heart-saving and cancer-protective benefits. In one survey, only 35 percent of women were aware of the connection between heart disease and menopause. Sixty-five percent of women do not have the proper knowledge to make educated decisions about the second half of their lives. They are in the dark, waiting for the light to shine in. I hope this book will throw the door open and let that light shine.

Estrogen use is a contraindication with active breast cancer. Medical literature confirms estrogen is safe and appropriate when administered five years after the initial Breast Cancer diagnosis. The medical literature demonstrates no increased risk of reoccurrence with estrogen use. In fact, there is a decreased incidence of recurrence with estrogen and an overall increased survival in estrogen users in comparison with those who do not take estrogen. But for women whose lives are severely impaired by estrogen deficiency, replacement is necessary. Let's approach these questions and concerns with care and a clear-minded understanding. When women express apprehension about taking estrogen, I lay all of the facts on the table. There is a slight risk of breast cancer with Premarin® and Provera® but not with estrogen alone. There is a dangerous risk of heart disease, osteoporosis, Alzheimer's and colon cancer without estrogen. A woman and her doctor must understand these risks, but most importantly make sure they understand all the facts of estrogen deficiency.

What Does This All Mean?

I'm advocating every woman should be on estrogen unless there is a contraindication. Your doctor should be able to educate you on natural hormone replacement. Perhaps this book will be the impetus for physicians to realize there are options. Perhaps this book will encourage physicians to take my comprehensive course on Natural Hormone Replacement. I am pleased to have been the originator of the most popular and the most successful HRT training course in the United States. Ultimately, it is my belief each physician should educate themselves and their patients on the most comprehensive health and lifestyle possible. Restoring hormone balance requires a partnership between each physician and patient. Please keep in mind, this is a journey. It is the process of finding out exactly what is right for you.

In Short…

Estrogen's Benefits: Protects against heart disease and stroke, decreases cholesterol, prevents and lowers the incidence of Alzheimer's Disease, improves memory, decreases symptoms of menopause, decreases insulin resistance, and prevents osteoporosis.

Estrogen's Side-Effects: In high doses, increased body fat, increased fluid retention, may cause headaches, may impair blood sugar metabolism, possible slight increased risk of strokes in older women who have pre-existing vascular disease and have never taken estrogen.

The Bottom Line: Estrogen happens to be the best tool to gear yourself up for the years to come. It builds bone, protects the heart, and stops Alzheimer's in its tracks. It has been proven to save many lives. Don't confuse natural bio identical hormones with synthetic hormones and don't extrapolate the harm of Premarin® and Provera® to natural bio identical estrogen. I urge you to open your eyes and reap the benefits.

Progesterone:
Estrogen's Natural Sidekick

Everyone in our office jokes about needing a
progesterone pill when they're in a bad mood.
It really does elevate your mood. Before, I felt
like I was on pins and needles every day. Now,
although I still have the daily stresses, I feel
better equipped to handle them. My PMS
symptoms are eliminated when I take
progesterone. I couldn't work or function the
week before my period. Now, there are no more
cramps, menstrual migraines, or mood swings.
I can't believe the difference it has made.

—Antonia, 48

If I forget to take my progesterone for a couple
of days all I do is cry and cry. It's amazing
how it influences my outlook on life. The side
effects and depression I experienced while on
Provera® are a thing of the past.

—Martha, 67

Estrogen replacement therapy was thought to be
working miracles on menopause until the early 1970s, when
researchers discovered that women on estrogen were
demonstrating an increased incidence of uterine bleeding.
Estrogen came with a high price most women were unwilling
to tolerate. Doctors and their patients shied away from
estrogen. Women were again faced with the arduous task of
balancing a normal life with the symptoms of menopause. Not

only did they miss out on estrogen's amazing ability to wipe out menopausal symptoms, but they failed to benefit from estrogen's heart healthy, bone building, and mood enhancing properties.

By prescribing estrogen alone, doctors were missing the fundamental tenet of total hormone replacement therapy: equilibrium. At optimal levels, hormones work in balance to ensure the body's successful battle against age-related disease. This is also true for the mind's ability to learn and retain information. The result of balancing hormones is the potential it gives us to live to a ripe old, healthy age!

This is the case for replacing both estrogen and progesterone. In early hormone replacement therapy, doctors and scientists did not recognize that the female body and sexuality are governed by two essential ovarian hormones, estrogen and progesterone.

Estrogen left alone will become dominant, resulting in excess estrogen side effects. Without progesterone's balancing properties, estrogen can become an adversary of the uterus. Problems such as uterine or endometrial cancer are due to excessive estrogen stimulation of uterine tissue. Youthful women are not prone to this problem because they produce plenty of progesterone, which provides a natural balance to estrogen. After menopause, women cease producing progesterone. This puts them at risk of estrogen dominance or over-stimulation of estrogen receptor sites. Researchers soon realized the importance of replacing progesterone along with estrogen. Natural balance was restored and resolved the problem of estrogen dominance or over-stimulation. As a natural hormone replacement patient, you will appreciate the many benefits of progesterone in your menopausal regimen. It can down-regulate receptor sites, hindering estrogen from over stimulating receptor sites in the breast and uterus, while providing other beneficial effects. All hormones are beneficial and need to be replaced to optimal, premenopausal levels.

Let's Get Technical: Progesterone and Gestation

Before I go any further with why you should be taking progesterone, you should understand progesterone's primary role as a gestational hormone. A woman's menstrual cycle is regulated through the action of two different hormones, estrogen and progesterone. Progesterone is produced in the corpus luteum, (the crater in the ovary, which is created as the egg emerges), the 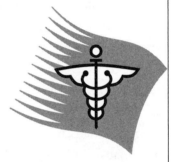 adrenal glands, and, during pregnancy, in the placenta. During the first half of a woman's monthly cycle, estrogen levels rise as the follicles in the ovaries prepare for ovulation. Progesterone levels rise during the second half of the cycle, preparing the uterine lining to accept the fertilized egg. If the egg is not fertilized, progesterone and estrogen levels drop and menstruation takes place. Progesterone levels are also important in creating a nourishing environment for a healthy pregnancy. Without enough progesterone, a woman has a difficult time carrying a baby full term. Progesterone stands for pro-gestational or the hormone of pregnancy. Progesterone maintains pregnancy, and if progesterone levels fall, a miscarriage occurs. Women who frequently miscarry are now prescribed natural progesterone to help maintain their pregnancy.

When a woman reaches her thirties, progesterone production begins to wane. After menopause, the levels plummet to almost zero. Unfortunately, menopause was originally seen as an estrogen-only deficiency and progesterone replacement therapy was considered unnecessary. When estrogen supplementation alone led to increased incidents of uterine bleeding, an abrupt and massive decline in estrogen replacement therapy took place. Progressive physicians went back to the drawing board for more research on the function of a woman's body. Doctors realized it is during and after menopause that progesterone works to promote feelings of vitality and health. Later on, a lack of progesterone can lead to some of the same problems as low levels of estrogen: osteoporosis, heart disease, a decrease in libido, and a significantly diminished quality of life. Estrogen and progesterone are necessary before, during and after menopause.

Progesterone should never be left out of your hormone regimen. Whether or not you have a uterus, studies demonstrate the importance of progesterone for a woman's health after menopause. Studies on progesterone are relatively new and we are learning more of the benefits as doctors and scientists more closely examine this previously overlooked hormone.

Ready to Get Off the Mood Swing?

One of my favorite comments from the women I treat with estrogen and progesterone is that they feel alive again. One woman in particular—we'll call her Felicia—used to call my practice quite often with complaint after complaint about things like hot flashes, night sweats, and insomnia. She was always abrupt, rude, and never had a nice thing to say about my staff or me. Finally, with much coercion, Felicia agreed to a trial 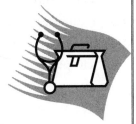 of natural hormones. Within a few weeks she called to thank me for taking away the huge weight she felt she had been lugging around for the last year. Her disposition and attitude completely changed. She even sent flowers to my staff. Her mood swings and depression resolved and her well being returned. No wonder her antidepressants were not working—her problem was not depression but a hormone deficiency. Returning her hormones to their optimal levels, as she stated, "Gave me my life back."

Progesterone has the amazing ability to act as an antidepressant, mild tranquilizer, and natural painkiller. It can be a tremendous treatment for premenstrual syndrome (PMS), helping to eliminate symptoms like moodiness, irritability, bloating, menstrual cramps, and headaches. These symptoms are often due to a fall in progesterone levels. The rapid fall in progesterone levels causes a withdrawal syndrome—a syndrome corrected only by replacing the hormone that is lacking. Many physicians prescribe antidepressants for PMS which may only result in slight improvement.

The key is to understand the deficiency and to replace it with just the right amount of the hormone. I have successfully treated hundreds of PMS patients by simply replacing their progesterone deficiency with natural progesterone. Natural progesterone can also eliminate the symptoms of menopause, including emotional instability, headaches, and mood swings. For women who are unable to take natural estrogen, natural progesterone can be prescribed to treat many of the common symptoms of menopause. This will help prevent some of the diseases associated with estrogen deficiency.

Around the time of menopause, women are experiencing major life changes. Children are going away to college or getting married. Marriages change and some couples find themselves adjusting to a new environment. To top it off, women are multi-taskers. They balance work with family and try to squeeze in a little time for themselves. Menopause can send this delicate balance reeling. Progesterone's natural calming effect can redirect menopausal depression. It enables women to wake in the morning refreshed for a new day.

The amount of sleep a person has influences mood and health. One of the most disrupting symptoms of menopause is sleep loss. Many patients complain they feel lethargic and apathetic during the day and anxious during the night. Progesterone has been shown to help eliminate sleeplessness, and I have observed this fact in my own patients. A 2001 study reported that women who took natural micronized progesterone reported significantly improved sleep over women taking the synthetic form of the hormone (Provera®). This is what the studies show—progesterone is tranquilizing while Provera® induces depression.

It is truly amazing how the body reacts to the sudden shift and decline of any hormone. Progesterone deficiency can cause minor to major complications. Replenishing these hormones prevents the complications. Mood and energy are only the icing on the cake when it comes to progesterone's awesome influence over the entire body.

Matters of the Heart

Statistics show that heart disease is the leading cause of death for women. Unfortunately, Provera® has been proven to negate some of estrogen's heart healthy benefits, and in turn has affected natural progesterone's reputation. Natural progesterone is rarely prescribed and instead women are taking Provera®—the synthetic and less effective replacement. The harmful effects of Provera® have led researchers to focus on how natural bio identical progesterone affects the heart. What they have learned is promising. So, let me clear up some misconceptions you may have encountered.

1. Provera® is not progesterone. The confusion comes in the terminology. The generic name for Provera® is medroxyprogesterone. However, many doctors and the medical literature chop off the medroxy portion of the name, referring to it as progesterone. They are two completely different molecules with completely different structures.

2. Bio identical progesterone is synergistic with estrogen to keep your heart working at youthful levels. It affects your lipids and protects against heart disease and stroke in a positive way. The process of plaque

91

formation involves cholesterol forming foam cells. These inflammatory cells cause plaque to develop inside blood vessels, leading to heart disease and stroke. Study after study has demonstrated estrogen and progesterone reduce foam cell formation and plaque buildup. The reverse is true of Provera®—it stimulates foam cell formation and plaque buildup. Estrogen and progesterone are synergistic with each other. Provera®, on the other hand, is antagonistic with estrogen, negating estrogen's beneficial effects on the heart.

When you were young, your heart was protected by estrogen and progesterone. With menopause, progesterone and estrogen levels decline at a rapid pace. As they decline, your heart loses protection. You've already read how estrogen works to keep the heart free of disease; but many people are unaware of how progesterone fits into the heart healthy equation.

Lipid metabolism is a determinant of heart health. It has been proven that estrogen has a positive effect on cholesterol. Studies now show that progesterone can also lower cholesterol and decrease the incidence of heart disease. In a German multi-center observational study, doctors monitored the efficacy and

> It has already been proven that estrogen has a positive effect on cholesterol. Studies are now showing that progesterone, too, can lower cholesterol and decrease the incidence of heart disease.

acceptance of two different regimens of postmenopausal hormone replacement therapies. The groups were separated by whether or not they took micronized progesterone continuously with natural estradiol or sequentially, days 16 through 25 of the monthly cycle. Both groups experienced considerable relief from menopausal symptoms. There was a reduction of cholesterol levels in both groups, but it was statistically more significant in the group using continuous progesterone therapy.

The landmark study, the Postmenopausal Estrogen/Progestin Interventions or PEPI Trial, also stressed the importance of natural progesterone over the synthetic version in relation to heart health. The results of this long-term study indicated that estrogen and estrogen plus natural progesterone provided the best results for lipid metabolism—increased HDL and lowered LDL levels.

Natural progesterone by no means replaces estrogen's heart healthy benefits. They are both synergistic and independently beneficial. Studies that have been done on primates have yielded promise for women seeking longer and more vital lives, including prevention of heart attacks.

Be selective when choosing your personal hormone replacement program. The synthetic form of progesterone, medroxyprogesterone acetate, or Provera®, has no protective effects for the heart. Medical studies now demonstrate that taking Provera® may actually be worse than no therapy at all. As far as the heart is concerned, they are right. On a positive note, medical studies now demonstrate natural progesterone enhances estrogen's ability to stave off heart disease. These studies have shown how progesterone enhances estrogen's beneficial effect on lipids, plaque formation, decrease in clotting (which causes heart attacks and strokes) and vasodilation.

Estrogen is the essential ingredient for a healthy heart. Natural progesterone enhances estrogen's effect on the body. This is important to understand because so many doctors have become comfortable prescribing Provera® in place of progesterone. Too many women are taking Provera® and increasing the risk of heart disease and stroke. I encourage you to take to heart the proven benefits of progesterone. If you are on estrogen and Provera®, please rethink exactly what you're trying to accomplish. You may be inhibiting the incidence of endometrial cancer, but also increasing your chance of heart complications with the use of Provera®. There is absolutely no reason to take Provera® when natural progesterone is readily available. Compounding pharmacies formulate and dispense progesterone that matches what your body normally produces. Natural progesterone not only protects against cancer, but also positively affects estrogen's impact on the heart.

Keeping these facts in mind, there is not really a choice. The medical literature provides overwhelming evidence of progesterone's protective effects and Provera's® harmful effects. With the influence of pharmaceutical marketing, physicians may still be ignorant of these facts. Natural progesterone suffers from lack of marketing, as do all natural hormones. They fall between the cracks and remain unnoticed. Many women find they end up educating their physicians, which ultimately benefits both patient and doctor.

Bone Up

Progesterone takes estrogen's powers for bone care one step further. Research has shown rather than simply preventing bone loss, progesterone can stimulate bone-building osteoblasts. In other words, progesterone may help build new bone. Our bones are under constant construction, being made and unmade, which is how they stay strong and healthy. When the bone-absorbing osteoclasts start outpacing the bone-building osteoblasts, our bones are left porous and susceptible to breakage.

Studies have shown how estrogen and progesterone affect both the biochemical markers of bone metabolism and bone mineral density. In a study featured in the journal, *Menopause*, researchers found that women supplementing with both estrogen and progesterone for a year had a significant bone mineral density **increase** in the lumbar spine and hipbone. They concluded that natural HRT favorably improved bone metabolism and prevented bone loss, while resulting in a slight increase of bone mineral density in the spine and hip.

Another study compared the bone mineral density of women who took hormone replacement therapy to that of women who did not. Researchers performed studies on paired bone biopsies obtained before and after two years of treatment. What they found is quite remarkable. Women on hormone replacement therapy displayed preservation of bone balance, while the women without HRT lost bone more quickly. The results of the tests illustrated that the hyperactivity of osteoclasts in the first phase of menopause can be quelled with a balanced hormone replacement regimen. This is prevention for osteoporosis and fractures.

All the studies cited above involve both estrogen and progesterone. Many researchers understand the delicate and essential balance between estrogen and progesterone. Estrogen is as important as progesterone to our aging clock, one gear meshes with the other for optimal function. Estrogen protects eyes, teeth, heart, bones, skin, vaginal tissue and lipids. Progesterone protects the uterus, bones, breasts, vaginal tissue, lipids and heart. When you lose the hormones you lose the protective effects.

There is one thing of absolute certainty—osteoporosis is a debilitating disease. Your risk of suffering from this disease can be greatly decreased through a balanced hormone replacement program. Again, I urge you to find a doctor who is aware of the changing times and treatment options available for menopause. A balanced combination of estrogen and progesterone is just the ticket to living a long and healthy life. Take that first step to healthy aging by ensuring you're on the right track with a complete natural hormone replacement program. There is no age limit for natural hormone replacement, as studies demonstrate positive effects of increasing bone density and fracture prevention for women in their seventies who have never taken hormones.

Since I Don't Have a Uterus, My Doctor Says I Don't Need Progesterone...

One of the most difficult aspects of being a doctor of preventative medicine is listening to the myths generated by people who should know better. Countless women have come to my office under the impression that they do not need progesterone if they do not have a uterus. The lack of a uterus does not negate the fact many other organs benefit from progesterone. Progesterone does so much more than just protect the uterus.

There are doctors who will argue over my use of an "unneeded" hormone in patients who have undergone hysterectomies. They were taught to believe—and as I once believed—that progesterone's role is solely to protect the uterus. If a woman doesn't have a uterus, she does not need progesterone. This may be the most impractical and unreasonable myth regarding hormone replacement therapy.

> To those women who no longer have a uterus, I emphasize this: your body now, as it has in the past, needs progesterone.

It is common practice for doctors to overlook the essential benefits progesterone offers for women who have had hysterectomies. To those women who no longer have a uterus, I emphasize: your body needs progesterone. You had it when you were younger and you will continue to need it in the years to come. There are progesterone receptors throughout the body that respond positively to progesterone stimulation.

The lack of progesterone can result in age-related disease, as readily as the lack of estrogen. Optimal levels of natural progesterone—levels that balance estrogen and progesterone—provide:

1. Proper bone density
2. Heart health

3. Lower cholesterol
4. Satisfactory quality of life
5. Contentment
6. Enhancement of estrogen's benefits
7. Protection against breast cancer and uterine cancer
8. Prevention of vaginal atrophy
9. Relief of PMS

Progesterone offers health benefits as well as feel-good benefits. Uterine health should follow heart health, bone density and emotional well-being—all reasons to prescribe natural progesterone. Progesterone also has far-reaching benefits on multiple organs. These benefits are often overlooked. Most physicians are only familiar with Provera® (medroxyprogesterone), which essentially offers no health benefits for women. To achieve complete and optimal health, you need both hormones in their natural form.

Synthetic vs. Natural

There is no doubt estrogen and progesterone protect women from many of the diseases that accompany aging. Post-menopausal women on estrogen/progesterone replacement therapy tend to lead a healthier lifestyle. Many of you have heard alarming stories about estrogen causing cancer and other negative side effects (breast tenderness, bloating, edema, bleeding and headaches) that may have left you wondering whether the benefits of estrogen replacement are all too good to be true.

Unfortunately, most of the estrogen and progesterone prescribed today is in the form of a synthetic. Premarin® and Provera®, the most popular form of hormones on the market, are good examples. Most of the purported harmful side effects of estrogen and progesterone arise from studies utilizing only these synthetic hormones.

Synthetic hormones are structurally different from human hormones and, as a result, they function differently from our natural hormones. Premarin® is made from the urine of pregnant mares. It contains more than ten different horse estrogens not found in the human body. These unnatural hormones account for the side effects and complications commonly ascribed to estrogen supplementation in women.

A natural hormone's structure is identical to the molecular structure of the hormone produced in the human body. It is only logical to replace a hormone with an identical match. There is no rhyme or reason behind replacing human estrogens with an estrogen that is chemically different.

We were taught in medical school the importance of maintaining the exact molecular structure of a hormone and receptor to assure the proper effect of the hormone. Why then are there synthetic hormones? Are they better? With all the side effects and complications, why are they even produced? A physician once asked me if natural hormones were as good as the synthetic hormones. I politely told him he had it backwards and reversed his question. One should ask—are any of the synthetic hormones as good as the natural hormones? The answer is emphatically "No".

Doctors were on the right track when they determined estrogen replacement needed the counterbalancing effects of its partner hormone, progesterone. However, instead of prescribing natural progesterone, they turned to what pharmaceutical companies had to offer: a synthetic progestin called Provera®. Provera® is as unnatural as it gets. In the late 1940's, it was devised in a test tube to look similar to progesterone, but it is definitely a distant relative. Progestins usually do more harm than good. In the *Physician's Desk Reference*, a good 60 percent of the text for Provera® is devoted to contraindications and adverse reactions. Instead of nullifying the effects of menopause, Provera® can cause:

1. Breast cancer
2. Depression
3. Weight gain
4. Blood clots in the lungs or brain
5. Water retention and bloating
6. Breast tenderness

The side effects sound worse than the actual effects of menopause. Despite documentation of the benefits of natural progesterone, most women today are still prescribed synthetic progestins. The benefits from progesterone supplementation are only achieved with natural progesterone and not with synthetic progestins. The only health benefit of Provera® is to protect the uterus. This is countered by many side effects, as well as risks of heart disease, stroke, breast cancer, or depression. Natural progesterone is just the opposite. It protects against heart disease, stroke, breast cancer and depression. All of this with virtually no side effects.

In a specific study, Hargrove et al. compared natural progesterone with that of medroxyprogesterone acetate (Provera®) in combination with estrogen therapy for menopausal women. They found that the women taking natural progesterone had more symptomatic improvement, an improved lipid profile, and they did not suffer from breakthrough bleeding or hyperplasia (build-up of endometrial cells in the uterus). The women reported no side effects but rather an enhanced quality of life and sense of well-being. Further, they wished to remain on this treatment beyond the end of the study. However, two women in the Provera® group requested to end their treatment early due to severe side effects.

Other studies have shown that the use of medroxyprogesterone (Provera®) can have some serious consequences on the female body, which are above and beyond the side effects listed in the *Physicians Desk Reference*. Many studies have concluded that synthetic hormone replacement therapy could be one of the root causes of breast cancer. Many women fear breast cancer and the possibility that hormone replacement therapy will only increase their risk. Natural, bio identical progesterone replacement is safe and effective without these risks.

The harmful effects of synthetic medroxyprogesterone (Provera®) are much more problematic than synthetic estrogen. More than 20 years of studies have well demonstrated the side effects of Provera®, taking up two full pages in the Physicians' Desk Reference. In contrast, the only side effect of natural progesterone is somnolence, or feeling sleepy. This is associated only with the oral form of progesterone and is alleviated by prescribing the dosage to be taken at night. A sublingual form of natural progesterone has no side effects!

It's strange how we, as a knowledgeable and conscientious society, weigh our options and our health. The Hargrove study is a perfect example of the effects of natural hormones. They were safe and effective, and women complied with their treatment. In fact, they wanted to continue even after the study ended. The Hargrove study took place in 1989, and nearly 20 years later, knowing the risk and side effects, doctors are still prescribing synthetic hormones. Cancer, depression, and general malaise are sidestepped when natural hormones are administered.

This is my advice: If you are handed a slip of paper with the prescription Premarin® or Provera® written on it, do not take it. Today, safer and more efficacious hormones are available. Bio identical, or natural hormones, provide all the benefits without the side effects. They are an exact match to the hormones your body produces naturally, and offer relief from bothersome menopausal symptoms. They also offer protection from the diseases that may interfere with living a long and prosperous life. A good rule of thumb is to always replenish your hormones with exactly what was there before. Replace the levels to what Hargrove et al. recommended. These are the levels of a younger, pre-menopausal woman.

I never advertise my practice because my patients, both in their appearance and their enthusiasm, spread the news like wildfire. Their new zeal for life makes them walking testaments of the benefits a patient can reap from natural hormone replacement therapy. The women above are only examples of the benefits hormone replacement can offer.

One of my patients, a 57-year-old woman we'll call "Grace," complained that not only had she gained the ten pounds that often accompany menopause, but she also had less energy and was suffering from bladder leakage due to decreased muscle strength. It was difficult for her to exercise, and when she did, she would often feel worse afterward. Her doctor prescribed synthetic estrogen and progestin but her symptoms worsened and she became depressed. Eventually she took herself off the synthetic hormones. Another physician tried another hormonal combination but this also made her feel worse and she quit that as well.

Finally, a mutual friend referred her to me. I started her on natural estrogen, progesterone, and testosterone. Within one month, she noticed vast improvement. The side effects she had experienced under her prior therapies were gone. She found she had improved strength and energy and saw a new person in herself. Her depression lifted, and she started her mornings with a desire to get up and go. And her husband was amazed at her revitalized interest in their sex life.

Another patient I worked with, a 49-year-old woman we'll call "Susan," was going through menopause and was prescribed synthetic hormones that she felt did not agree with her body. In addition to feeling the hot flashes and mood swings associated with menopause, she felt that her health and energy had deteriorated as well. She no longer felt alive. Susan had asked her private physician to prescribe natural hormones. He merely stated that he had been using what he called "natural" hormones for the past 20 years and had had no complications.

Like many of my patients, her friends referred her to my office where we worked out a balanced prescription of natural hormones. After a matter of weeks, she called, excited to report the dramatic results. Susan stated that she was amazed with how quickly her menopausal symptoms had subsided, and her overall sense of well-being improved. She has been so excited about the results of natural hormones that she is eagerly telling her friends.

The Challenge

Any woman who feels suspended in menopause needs to know there is more to life. Any woman who wants to get the most out of her years to come now has options. Do what thousands of women have already done: embrace life with both hands and mold it into the shape and length you want. You no longer have to flounder through menopause and beyond. There is nothing more important than improving quality of life through natural hormone replacement. There is no mystery behind the benefits and protection of natural hormone replacement therapy — you're only supplying your body with natural tools to maintain a healthy and happy life. Medical advances have extended the *quantity* of years; I'm working on extending the quality.

Natural progesterone and estrogen are essential to all women. Do not jeopardize the protection they offer against heart disease, stroke, cancer, osteoporosis, and Alzheimer's disease. Give them a chance—they will improve your skin, mood, sex life and self-image. Make your 40's, 50's, 60' and beyond the best years of your life.

In Short...

Progesterone Benefits: Progesterone works with estrogen to relieve menopausal symptoms, protect against breast and uterine cancer, prevent osteoporosis, improve heart health, and enhance overall feelings of well-being. For pre-menopausal women, progesterone eliminates

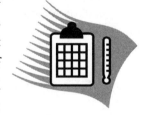

---

painful menstrual cramps, mood swings, heavy bleeding, dysphoria, bloating, and menstrual migraines.

Progesterone Side-Effects: Natural progesterone has no harmful side effects. If taken in oral form, it can cause some sleepiness.

Bottom Line: Natural progesterone, used in conjunction with estrogen, provides women, with or without a uterus, significant relief to many of the symptoms associated with aging and menopause. There are many health benefits as well as feel-good benefits.

Estrogen, Progesterone and Cancer
What's the Real Story

The relationship of hormones to cancer is complex and defies simple statements. Many hormones discussed in this book are misunderstood because the cancer issue is also misunderstood. When you throw in the use of synthetic hormones, the topic gets even more confusing.

Most physicians are unaware of the recent literature demonstrating that progesterone protects against breast cancer. This literature emphasizes the higher the level of progesterone, the greater the protection against breast cancer. In the traditional medical community you will hear that progesterone provokes cancer. Many physicians make this statement because they mistake progesterone for medroxyprogesterone (progestin). The names are similar but their structures, physiology and side effects are completely different.

We should review which hormones protect the body and which ones are detrimental to the body. Again, from an evolutionary standpoint, the body does not make anything harmful to itself. All organisms will adapt to their environment for survival. Cholesterol is the source of our hormones, digestive juices, and is an antioxidant, all of which are beneficial. Cholesterol is not harmful until it becomes oxidized or damaged. The same applies to our hormones. They are beneficial to our bodies; they do not harm us. It is only when we change the chemical structure, including oxidized cholesterol, that hormones and cholesterol become harmful.

Let's Get Technical

The P53 gene blocks growth of breast cancer cells by destroying cancer cells. Stimulation or up regulation of the BCL2 gene promotes the growth of cancer cells that is offset by stimulation of P53 gene. The P53 gene blocks formation of cancer. Maximum expression of the P53 gene is found at mid-menstrual cycle when progesterone levels peak, and during pregnancy when serum levels are very high. When 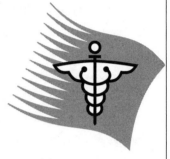 progesterone levels are low, other genes increase their cellular responses, which provoke breast stimulation.

This is the exact mechanism by which progesterone protects against breast stimulation and breast cancer formation.

On the other hand, medroxyprogesterone blocks progesterone receptor sites and prevents progesterone attachment to the receptor site, thereby allowing breast stimulation. Medroxyprogesterone increases the risk of breast cancer eight to nine times over baseline by simply blocking progesterone. Thus it can be interpreted as anti-progesterone. How inappropriate that the chemical medroxyprogesterone even contains the name progesterone, as it is a progesterone antagonist, not promoter! Only natural progesterone molecules kill cancer cells and at the same time stimulate the P53 gene, which in turn stops the spread of breast cancer cell lines.

Progesterone also stimulates the breast cancer resistance protein (BCRP). There is a balance between estrogen and progesterone and BCRP expression. This demonstrates why progesterone is so very important in post-menopausal women. Estrogen has many health benefits, yet some of these effects might be problematic if not balanced by progesterone. The incidence of breast cancer dramatically increases at menopause. Since women lose their hormones at menopause, why is there a surge in breast cancer with loss of estrogen? Obviously, estrogen has nothing to do with this. Scientific literature now demonstrates that the loss of progesterone and its associated breast cancer protective proteins results in this surge in breast cancer at menopause.

The most powerful medical study to date, the Women's Health Initiative trial, proved that estrogen alone did not increase risk of cancer. On the other hand, progesterone stimulates the growth and spread of BCRP. However, both estrogen (estradiol) and progesterone increase BCRP production more than progesterone alone! The mechanism is complex, but well documented. A recent article published in *Circulation* (April 2007) demonstrated an increase in breast cancer with Premarin® and Provera®. The use of estradiol and progesterone demonstrated no increase in cancer. This is another study that should be in the headlines of every newspaper.

Progesterone has also been shown to protect against breast cancer growth by activating P27 gene promoters which cause cancer cell apoptosis (the killing of cancer cells). Research has demonstrated several mechanisms by which progesterone protects against cancer.

Medroxyprogesterone, on the other hand, has been shown to increase cancer cell production and growth by acting in the opposite manner as progesterone. What this tells us is that cancer seems to be provoked primarily because of a *lack* of progesterone or the presence of a progestin (Provera®) and not necessarily due to any effect of estrogen.

Instead of headlines claiming that estrogen is dangerous, the headlines should read, "Estrogen is not dangerous: breast cancer is induced by lack of progesterone or the use of medroxyprogesterone and not due to estrogen.

Another common misconception surrounds the use of the term "estrogen-sensitive cancer." Once a cancer forms, receptor sites develop on the tumor. These receptor sites might be stimulated by estrogen, which might cause the cancer to grow. This is why doctors avoid treating women who have breast cancer with estrogen. In fact, doctors commonly prescribe Tamoxifen or Armidex®, which are estrogen blockers. These chemotherapeutic agents block the binding or production of estrogen to prevent growth of the tumor by estrogen stimulation.

However, this does not mean estrogen causes the cancer to form in the first place! The Women's Health Initiative proved a decrease in breast cancer when estrogen alone was used. Although many women might believe estrogen-receptors with positive tumors are caused by estrogen, this is simply not true. It only means as the cancer grows, it develops receptor sites that become sensitive to estrogen. Estrogen does not cause.

Let's Get Technical

There are many mechanisms by which a breast cancer can develop. There is an interplay of many genes, antiproliferative proteins and stimulatory proteins. Environmental agents might stimulate genes that cause increased expression of breast cancer growth proteins in peri-menopause. Loss of progesterone or the administration of cancer-causing progestins increases growth of stimulatory proteins. Loss of

---

progesterone in menopause decreases the protective proteins of the P53 gene. This probably accounts for the increase in breast cancer that occurs after menopause. Thus it is not estrogen, but the loss of progesterone that puts women at risk for cancer.

The bottom line is:

- Estrogen does not cause cancer.
- Progestins tend to provoke cancer.
- Progesterone protects against cancer.

Hormones are the body's friends. Their disappearance causes the body to deteriorate and become unhealthy. Replenishing the body with natural hormones will help it become healthy again. If we want to be healthy, we have to give back to our bodies the hormones that make it thrive.

Testosterone:
Revitalize Every Aspect of Your Life!

What a piece of work is a man.
—from William Shakespeare's *Hamlet*

While this chapter deals with men and hormones, every woman should read and educate themselves about how to maintain health, happiness, and well being in their spouse

Once there was a man who had spent his life jumping hurdles and cunningly climbing social and political ladders. His ambition had built an economical empire and his decisions trickled down into many aspects of other people's lives; when he moved it seemed people held their breath so as not to disturb him. He held all the strings, and with one tug could send a person's world toppling down. 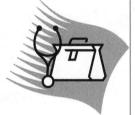 This sounds appealing to many men, this powerful resonance that engulfs a man's surroundings. But do you know that this man also succumbed to a mid-life crisis? As with most men suffering andropause, he was ignorant of the symptoms of his age-related hormone deficiency. He had never heard either within or outside of his social circles that men suffered, like women, a sort of menopause.

Like many men, this hormone alteration presented itself in the disguise of fatigue and disinterest in life. Instead of being vibrant and motivated, he lost his ambition and drive. The awesome director was losing his ability to lead and encourage as he once did. He now became tired and withdrawn, with no energy or desire to exercise or travel. His wife noticed that his libido and performance had declined. The romantic lover he used to be was only a memory.

or significant other. This chapter starts with a story as I believe stories paint pictures, and pictures speak a thousand words...

You may be saying to yourself, "C'mon, is this guy for real?" The story may sound stereotypical, but stereotypes come into being for a reason. With the decline of hormones every aspect of a person's health and well-being is affected. We work hard to finally feel comfortable in our own bodies and after 50 years, we're assaulted with a whole new setting. A decrease in testosterone accounts for the loss of a man's sense of well-being. Testosterone replacement will allow a successful transition into the rest of his adulthood. By the time a man reaches 50, we see a significant drop in his testosterone levels. Unfortunately for many men, this slow but sure decline has not been an issue of discussion. As with the example of the man above, ignorance does not always bring bliss.

I've seen testosterone work wonders for a man's ego. It has helped marriages waning under sexual dysfunction and depression. Many men and women are uneducated about andropause, or male menopause. The whole idea of men going through menopause and needing hormone replacement therapy can be emasculating. Virility is second nature to a man. Starting when hormonal changes occur around age 40, men see a marked decline in abilities they once perceived to be as easy as breathing. Men find that erections are not as frequent, sex is not as exciting, ejaculation is not as powerful, and the stamina and endurance they once experienced has diminished. It seems that after 45, men often have a hard time rising for any occasion. This is what is referred to as andropause, male menopause or viropause. So why do most men not know anything about andropause? Andropause has recently received attention and recognition, but why the holdup? There are many reasons behind the stifling of its discovery along with many frames of mind that are still hindering its cure.

Slipping Into Lower Gear

Men are blasted with a reality check during their mid-40s. Their hormone levels drop and the erection that once greeted them in the morning ceases. Muscle definition fades and men get flabby around the middle. "It's all a matter of aging," they're told, when in actuality, doctors should find it easy to diagnose andropause or hypogonadism. Once a man awakens in the morning without an erection, he has hypogonadism. In addition, there are other ways men recognize they have andropause. When men start worrying about whether they will stay hard throughout sex, they have it. When men are fearful of having sex without popping Viagra, they have it. When men hope they would again have that strong intense orgasm, they have it. Men don't talk about these things, but they all know something is not right. Most men prefer to never stop testosterone once they start using it. This is living proof of what I'm alluding to. Recent studies have well demonstrated that when Viagra doesn't work, the trick is to just add testosterone.

Testosterone is truly a life source to the male body. Highly specialized leydig cells in the testes produce 90 to 95 percent of testosterone. A small amount is produced by the adrenal glands. Testosterone travels though the body via the bloodstream and binds to receptors on target tissues, which then trigger the required response. There are testosterone receptors throughout the body, including important areas of the brain. Testosterone is the defining factor in a male's development. It's the flipped switch that, during puberty, sends boys reeling with the changes in their emotions and physical appearance. At this time, testosterone triggers the growth of pubic hair, facial hair, deepening of the voice and the general appearance of a more masculine body shape.

For many years, endocrinologists believed testosterone levels were not affected by age. Only recently have doctors detected and proven an age-related testosterone decline. Endocrinologists did not believe testosterone took a dip after 45, because they were measuring the wrong type of testosterone. They measured the total amount of testosterone rather than focusing on free testosterone. Much of a man's testosterone is tied up or bound to a protein called sex hormone-binding globulin (SHBG). Once bound to SHBG, the testosterone is no longer obtainable by the rest of the body. There is only a small amount (about 4 percent) of bio-available or free testosterone accessible to the body. Research has shown free testosterone becomes more bound with age, leaving readily available levels of testosterone low while total testosterone levels remain normal. This is where one of the biggest hang-ups has occurred and why symptoms of aging were not tied to a testosterone decline. Only when doctors and scientists honed in on the bio-available testosterone did they realize there was a definite decline. It is the fall in bio-available or free testosterone that is responsible for the signs and symptoms of andropause.

Total vs. Free Testosterone—There is a Difference

In the previous section, I mentioned the difference between total testosterone and free testosterone. The total testosterone level is much greater than the free testosterone, as most of testosterone exists in the blood as a protein-bound complex. It serves as the carrier or transport molecule that stores and sends testosterone throughout the body. This transport protein tightly binds testosterone, making it difficult for testosterone to float freely in the blood. Liken this total testosterone to money in the bank—it's yours but you don't have access to it, as it is stored in the bank. The free testosterone, on the other hand, floats freely in the blood and is available to be used and attach to testosterone receptor sites. Liken this to money in your pocket—it can be used right now.

As men age, they lose their free testosterone, which is the most important testosterone. Even though the total testosterone remains normal, free testosterone levels fall with age. This is due to increased amounts of the protein that binds testosterone. SHBG increases because of many factors. The cause most noted in the medical literature is elevation of estrogen. Although estrogen might have a small influence, it is minimal. This fact is often misunderstood when there is not a clear understanding of the physiology of estrogen. In women, oral estrogen passes through the liver and results in increased SHBG. However, transdermal estrogen does not increase SHBG. Since men do not take oral estrogen, the serum level of estrogen in men does not account for much elevation of SHBG. Typically SHBG increases secondary to age, alcohol use, obesity, lack of exercise and medications.

The elevation of SHBG and resultant decrease in free testosterone can be remedied either by lowering SHBG levels or by administering testosterone. Raising the free testosterone levels into a more optimal range may result in a concomitant high, super-physiologic level of total testosterone. Total testosterone levels can increase by two to three times the normal levels. When patients and their physicians encounter extremely high levels, they may fear that these high levels are harmful. They are not at all harmful, and in fact are most beneficial. Remember, our goal is to raise hormone levels to the optimal range of a young adult for free testosterone. We do not treat the total testosterone level. This level is meaningless with a Natural Hormone Replacement Program. If the physician and patient are not experienced and knowledgeable in the science behind optimal hormone replacement, this level will be meaningless and misdiagnosed.

Another important point is the difference between optimal and normal. Normal for one's age is not *optimal* for one's age. The medical literature supports replacement levels to that of a younger age, typically 20 to 30 years old. At these levels, optimal health is attained, as well as the feel-good effects. The problem is how one defines normal and optimal. Normal for a 70-year-old is not normal for a 20-year-old. If a 20- year-old man has the testosterone level of a 70-year-old man, he will not feel well. If a 70-year-old man has the level of a 70-year-old man, this is considered normal. No man should have the testosterone level of a 70-year-old as supported in our medical literature. In reality we are not trying to be 30; however our goal is to optimize levels to those we would see in a 20 to 30 year-old. A free testosterone lab value of 25 may be interpreted as optimal when in fact this level is quite low. A lab value of 40 would be interpreted as being too high when in reality it is a perfect level and our goal for a younger person. All the medical studies utilize hormone dosages resulting in levels on the upper end of the physiologic range. These are levels found in young adults.

In past years, various labs would list the testosterone ranges for all ages next to the lab results. Today, the labs publish only the normal levels based on a person's age. This does not provide the appropriate indication of *optimal* levels as it is age specific. For example, normal free testosterone levels for a 60-year-old man range from 5 to 25. Optimal is therefore expected to be 25. A traditional medical doctor would interpret 25 as optimal. But remember, our goal is to replace free testosterone levels to that of a younger male. These free testosterone levels would be 30 to 40. A lab value of 40 would be interpreted by the lab as being too high, when in reality the level of 40 is perfect and is always our goal.

Balancing Act: The Testosterone-Estrogen Ratio

Doctors and scientists have been researching the male endocrine system for the last several decades. Their research has discovered multiple reasons to correct and prevent andropause. I've read countless articles, participated in a myriad of discussions, and found many people are now coming to understand the importance of preventing andropause. All the medical literature now supports the importance of preventing the deterioration associated with andropause, both for health reasons and for quality of life.

How do we achieve optimal levels of testosterone? Simply by replacing it. Testosterone supplementation does increase estrogen levels and SHBG. SHBG may cause a slight decrease in free testosterone availability. The treatment is to increase testosterone supplementation until free testosterone levels are optimal. I do not recommend lowering estrogen levels, as this will lead to the harmful effects of low estrogen. During the past 40 years, hundreds of testosterone studies have shown increased estrogen levels in men are not harmful. Testosterone supplementation always increases serum estrogen (estradiol) levels. If indeed the increase in estrogen among men was harmful, based on hundreds of studies throughout the last 50 years, it would have been revealed. Every study has shown testosterone to be beneficial and not harmful. Therefore, we must assume since testosterone always raises estrogen, estrogen is also beneficial.

There are over 20 medical studies demonstrating low estrogen levels in men are harmful and raising estrogen levels is beneficial. Optimal estrogen levels are necessary for adequate bone growth, osteoporosis prevention, dementia, Alzheimer's and heart disease. If a man wishes to increase the risk of these problems, keep estrogen levels low, if you get my drift. Despite all the claims in the neutraceutical literature, no one has been able to show me any study demonstrating increased estrogen levels are harmful in the presence of optimal testosterone. The medical literature only demonstrates beneficial effects. I do not recommend anyone lower their serum estrogen levels. It is actually the testosterone/estrogen ratio that is most important. Loss of testosterone and increase of estrogen results in estrogen blocking testosterone receptor sites. The simple solution is to raise testosterone levels back to optimal levels, thereby reducing the effect from estrogen. The impression that estrogen is harmful is unfounded. Estrogen is not harmful. It is the loss of testosterone which results in a disproportionate ratio of testosterone to estrogen which is responsible for the side effects. Once this ratio is corrected using testosterone replacement, estrogen becomes quite beneficial.

It's amazing that almost 38 years ago we put a man on the moon, we can split the atom and we can exchange a diseased human heart for a new one. We have made medical and technological leaps but are still mystified by the inner workings of male biology. We're finding one obstacle after another, and the truth is we got a late start. I hope every man reads this chapter and recognizes that as his body systems retire and he begins to feel "old", he is not alone. Most of all, I hope this will encourage every man to seek the available options that will change the quality of his life. You must find a physician knowledgeable about testosterone replacement and a physician willing to prescribe to optimal levels.

Foremost, your physician must understand optimal replacement and the difference between normal and optimal. The medical literature supports raising testosterone levels to the upper level of normal. This provides protection against heart disease, diabetes and loss of muscle strength. In addition optimal levels boost libido, energy, motivation, cognition and memory. Most physicians will interpret low normal levels as perfectly fine. Normal for your age means you are just as low as everyone else your age. Normal is definitely not optimal—normal is detrimental to your health and well-being. The normal level for middle age is the level where men fall apart. Every medical study on testosterone utilizes a dose which raises testosterone levels to the upper normal range for a young adult.

A physician skilled in HRT understands normal is exactly where you do not want to be. Two of our most prestigious medical studies have demonstrated the higher the testosterone level, (within the optimal range) the more protected you are against heart disease, diabetes, elevated cholesterol and the many other problems associated with middle age. Optimal is exactly where everyone should be. This applies to all hormones, not just testosterone.

Up until now this chapter has focused on the importance of men and their physicians educating themselves about natural hormone replacement. It has been my experience that 75 percent of the men I see have been dragged into my practice by their wives. It is usually the women who are knowledgeable about hormones from their own personal research. Women should take note of this chapter, so they can better understand how to keep the men in their lives healthy.

The Ultimate Aphrodisiac

We now know that 60 percent of all men by the age of 65 have abnormally low levels of testosterone. The remaining 40 percent will have low normal levels, which are sub-optimal. We also know that testosterone levels are directly linked to a man's sex drive. It is not a coincidence that when boys go through puberty, their sexual awareness soars. Nor is it by chance that this awareness dulls into a frustrated indifference during a man's mid-40s to early 50s. The sexual prowess a man was once proud of becomes a sporadic and less passionate visitor. For men with a low level of testosterone, the decline is acute. Many of my male patients come to my practice after suffering for years in silence. They have tiptoed around their symptoms and have a hard time looking me in the eye. They wait for me to make an educated guess—their sex drive is at an all-time low. You can't imagine the dismay on their face when I tell them this is normal. Their dismay quickly dissipates when I let them in on the best kept secret—there is a solution.

One of my patients—we'll call him Sean -- was 58 when he finally came to visit me. What prompted his visit is a great story, which sadly begins with a tragedy. Sean had lost his wife to cancer and after two years had met an attractive woman 20 years his junior whose company he enjoyed immensely. Although they were compatible in most aspects of their companionship, he felt he lacked the 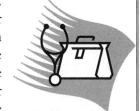 passion and adventure she desired under the covers. He had become accustomed to the infrequent lovemaking he and his wife shared during the last years of their marriage, and this new pressure made him frustrated and embarrassed at his lack of sexual appetite. He felt rusty and awkward. His friends and general practitioner basically advised him to take it easy, that he was no longer expected to perform sexual acrobatics, and that this was what old age was all about. Sean felt guilty that he couldn't keep up with his female friend and decided he should end their six-month relationship.

Luckily, he ran into an old college buddy of his who was a current patient of mine. Over coffee they began to compare notes about their social lives and found that they had a few similarities. They were both dating younger women. Yet, his friend spoke of the experience with excitement and optimism. His friend shared his secret, and Sean soon made an appointment to visit me.

Sean's problem was not hard to decipher. His testosterone levels were quite low. We designed the perfect dose to meet his needs and after two months, Sean and his fiancée began experiencing an exciting life beyond and in spite of what society calls "old age." He told me it felt like someone rewound his life a full 20 years and pushed play again. His fiancée also wrote me a letter, thanking me for the freshness that "whatever I did" added to their relationship. "He's so much more playful and alive now." Sometimes I chuckle to myself, thinking that perhaps one day she'll be straining to keep up with him. However, if this woman is over 40, then she needs to read the chapter on testosterone for women in order to keep up with him!

Sean's story is just one confirmation of how testosterone supplementation can enhance the quality of a man's sex life. There are many documented studies illustrating the same positive outcome. Most men have a hard time owning up to sexual dysfunction. Men's sex lives define who they are. When a man begins to feel a decrease in his sexuality, he may undergo an identity crisis, better known as a mid-life crisis. I would like to insert a little cautionary disclaimer: since sexuality is such a dynamic part of our character, there are certain facets that affect sexuality which testosterone cannot help. Testosterone cannot help a man who suffers from psychological problems or clinical depression.

As the gradual decline of testosterone begins, supplementation is just the spice to heat up a man's sex life. Some studies have shown testosterone affects the nerves and skeletal muscles involved in erections. We're still unsure of the exact workings, but it is obvious in studies and in the testimonies of patients that testosterone can get the gears working properly again. Not only that, but testosterone can rev up a sluggish and listless sex drive. It increases sensation, and improves orgasm and overall satisfaction. A low testosterone level not only creates mechanical problems but it also affects an overall outlook on sex. So many of my patients say they "just don't feel like it" or they're "too tired." After a few months of testosterone supplementation, these same men feel a sudden zest in their sex lives.

Improving Your Emotional State

Our emotional stance in life can directly influence every action or reaction we have. I've seen in more than one instance how depression can totally change a man's life. Because men are not well versed in this natural phase in their life, they do not recognize the signs and cannot seek out the proper channels for help. What I have noticed in my practice is that many men who suffer depression and moodiness have low-normal levels of testosterone. With the proper dosage, these men come alive again. They're more assertive, which motivates success in their careers and in their personal lives.

Many studies reinforce testosterone's reputation as being the feel-good hormone that pulls men out of the mid-life rut. Hypogonadism and low-normal levels of testosterone impair a man's sexual ability, and also seem to fog his perception of life. Low testosterone levels are linked to both sexual dysfunction and despondency. Testosterone has shown itself to be a strong ally to a man's ego and sex drive. It not only improves a man's mood but it puts him in the mood.

One of my patients, 50-year old "Greg," was referred to my clinic by his psychiatrist. After almost a year of sampling different antidepressants and finding no positive results, Greg was directed to my office for a complete hormone deficiency evaluation.

He confided that the antidepressants were killing his sex drive, and in the heat of the moment, he couldn't get or maintain an erection. The antidepressants did not work and made his depression worse. He expressed that it was increasingly difficult to concentrate at work and he had a hard time attending to assignments formerly awarded to him for his ability to be quick and concise. The thought of exercise overwhelmed him. By the time he got home from work at night, he was exhausted from just thinking of all the things he needed to accomplish.

I put Greg on a hormone regimen, including testosterone. Within one month, Greg did an about-face. His antidepressants no longer had ill effects on his sex life (because he no longer needed them). After an additional month, he had the fire and drive to again accomplish assignments at work. His relationship with his wife got the boost it needed, both sexually and emotionally. The prescription of hormone replacement therapy completely turned his life around. His mental clarity sharpened and he's full of the get-up-and-go and optimism he thought he had lost along with his 30s.

Often, what comes across as depression may in reality be the effects of low testosterone levels. Unfortunately, these symptoms are diagnosed as depression and treated with antidepressants. Depression is usually not the cause of the problem. For men with true psychological depression which responds only to antidepressant medicine, there are often sexual side effects. The treatment that relieves the effects of

SSRIs is testosterone. Men and women who have been prescribed SSRIs should put their fears aside, as testosterone easily reverses the sexual side effects of antidepressants.

Lose That Middle!

The word "testosterone" suggests an image of something rugged, rough and aggressive—something that makes men, men. When someone says the word "steroid" the image suddenly changes to illegal. We immediately think of the darkened reputation of sportsmanship and drugs that can seriously impede the health of its user. Unfortunately, these last few images have put a damper on testosterone's good name. Since the 1950's, synthetic anabolic steroids were employed by athletes to enhance their physical performance. These anabolic steroids increase muscle bulk and shorten the recovery time after a strenuous workout. There are people who misuse anabolic steroids for muscle-enhancing and fat-trimming benefits. As the result of pressure from professional sports and bodybuilding competitions, many athletes abuse harmful steroids to add that extra push. That extra push can sometimes cause some serious consequences. Young athletes abusing synthetic anabolic steroids are in danger of sterility, liver damage, cancer and even death. One must not equate synthetic anabolic steroids with testosterone. Testosterone is not a synthetic anabolic steroid, it is a bio identical hormone with many health benefits for both men and women.

Most young men have normal levels of testosterone and their use of synthetic anabolic steroids is inappropriate. Middle-aged men with low levels of testosterone develop health issues from lack of testosterone. Therefore, treating hormone deficiencies in middle-aged men should not be compared to the abuse of synthetic agents by young athletes. The synthetic anabolic agents cause numerous problems not seen with natural testosterone replacement. Again, natural testosterone is healthy and beneficial and should not be compared to the synthetic, anabolic steroids.

As a healthy man ages, he begins to grow around the middle. Men usually fall victim to central or visceral obesity, also known as the "pot belly," the "beer gut," or the "spare tire." Most men joke about their growing stomach, but there is nothing funny about the risks associated with adding on the inches. This spare tire increases a man's risk of cardiovascular disease or type II diabetes. As men take on the battle of the bulge, muscle melts into fat and exercise seems to become a feat of will power and ability. Most of my male patients joke about their belly using humor to deal with the changing shape of their body.

One of my patients had tried everything from stepping up his workout regimen to virtually starving himself. The spare tire was absolutely resistant to all his efforts. One day, Frank happened upon an advertisement for a lecture I was giving and decided he might need to listen to what I had to say. A few days after the lecture, he made an appointment to see me in my practice. We quickly determined his testosterone levels were low. I prescribed testosterone cream and after several months Frank's testosterone was restored to optimal levels. His belly did a disappearing act as his body became firmer and more defined. He told me he didn't ever remember looking and feeling this good. He had lost body fat and gained muscle as if he were 30 again.

Study after study confirms testosterone's powerful influence over the masculine figure. With the decline of testosterone, men put on the pounds and sluggishly haul them around. But here's the good news. There is no reason to settle into your oversized body and accept your spare tire. Fat-to-muscle ratio increases because your testosterone decreases. Your energy levels decline, your mood levels dwindle and you lose muscle and gain fat. With the supplementation of testosterone, a man has the stamina to be a husband, father, professional and sportsman late into his life. It's amazing what a small amount of testosterone will do for a man's self image and strength. No man is too old for hormone therapy.

Out with the Old, In with the New

Without the proper maintenance of our muscles or the continual remodeling of our bones, our bodies will collapse.

> **As the life span in men increases and baby boomers add years to their lives, bone fractures in men are expected to double by the year 2025.**

Some of the most powerful tools in keeping the body in prime shape are hormones. Optimal hormone levels are the key that allows the body to be built to last.

As men pass through andropause, the risk of osteoporosis increases. Most men consider this debilitating disease a female frailty. The truth is, men become just as susceptible when their testosterone levels sink below normal. As the life span in men increases and baby boomers add years to their lives, bone fractures in men are expected to double by the year 2025. Muscles support bone while bone supports the body. As we age, both the insulating muscles and the bones they wrap around get weaker and weaker.

Let's Get Technical: Sex Hormones and Our Bones

Sex hormones have been the main focus of bone deterioration. Researchers have found they directly influence and regulate the osteoclasts, the cells that remove old bone, and osteoblasts, the cells that create new bone. Both estrogen and testosterone foster a compatible and symbiotic liaison between the two juxtaposed cellular structures of osteoblasts and osteoclasts. The rate of osteoclast and osteoblast genesis depends on the presence of testosterone. Testosterone has been shown to help this process remain equalized.

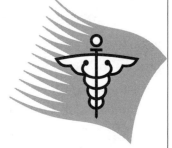

Studies have shown that hypogonadal men experience bone loss. They have an increased risk of hip fracture, and without testosterone, it seems, their bones whittle away. As early as 1948, testosterone administration was shown to reduce fracture occurrence.

Supplementation of calcium and vitamin D along with a good exercise regimen are required for bone formation and prevention of bone loss. The basis for their inclusion in bone creation is hormonal. Estrogen eliminates gross percentages of bone loss in women. Preliminary studies have shown testosterone administration accomplishes the same results in men.

Testosterone doubles or triples bone density in comparison with estrogen. In a recent study, the longest of its kind, it was demonstrated that all supplements together, including calcium, vitamin D, and bisphosphonates (e.g. Fosamax® and Actonel®), still resulted in significant bone density loss year after year. The only treatment that increased bone density was estrogen. And just imagine, testosterone is three times stronger than estrogen.

Men with low testosterone have a decrease in energy. They find it next to impossible to expend what they do have at the gym. Bones need weight-bearing exercise to grow in mass and strength. Without it, they deteriorate. Therefore, the lack of testosterone creates a double-edged sword. If you don't have enough testosterone, your bones suffer the consequences. As men reach 50 they often do not have enough energy to physically endure the weight-bearing exercise which can alter the downward spiral.

It may come as a surprise, but researchers have determined that it is the conversion of testosterone into estrogen that is responsible for most bone growth. Studies show that blocking testosterone causes bone loss. Administering estrogen alone reverses the bone loss. This is another perfect example of estrogen's positive effect in males and proof we should never lower estrogen in men.

Testosterone is just another hormone your aging body finds hard to produce. This hormone is packed with a vigorous punch. You only have one body, so it is worth choosing the right tools to build it to last. Testosterone, along with a diet designed for your bones and a little sweat of the brow, could help your body last far into its 90s. Testosterone therapy is a choice worth making, no bones about it.

What it Really Means to Have a Good Heart

Statistics are grim when it comes to men and heart disease. The American Heart Association estimates that 90,000 men between the ages of 45 and 64 die each year from heart attacks or other heart complications. Ninety thousand is a tremendous number of people who more likely than not could have prevented the onset of heart disease. Optimal levels of testosterone create a healthy environment to protect against all aspects of heart disease. Hormones are the essential building blocks for a healthy and vibrant lifestyle. As I explained in the estrogen chapter, women find themselves facing a new set of risks in the years after menopause. Their hormones plummet and they feel awful as they experience an actual physical deterioration. The same happens with men and low testosterone levels. In the case of testosterone, absence does not make the heart grow fonder. Therefore, it's safe to say testosterone and the heart are closely related. This is a prime example of how one hormone can make or break an organ, in this case, the heart.

Unfortunately, this fact has been overlooked. For a while, researchers actually believed testosterone was bad medicine for the heart. Scientists thought this explained why women avoided heart problems up into their 60s while their male counterparts were dropping like flies from heart attacks. Researchers believed that estrogen saved the heart while testosterone was a traitor to the same body that produced it. Nothing could be further from the truth. Normal to high levels of testosterone have been proven to increase a male's life span by decreasing the incidence of heart disease. Higher levels of testosterone decrease overall cholesterol levels while maintaining HDL at optimal levels. The measure of HDL, our good cholesterol, is a positive indicator of heart health. With testosterone boosting HDL to proper levels, the heart is safe from illness. Beyond this, testosterone has an artery-dilating effect, which increases coronary blood flow. Statins, the most commonly prescribed heart medicine, offer none of these benefits.

> I've had several male patients who complain to me of chest pain. "Roy" said it felt like a vise had a hold of his heart and someone kept cranking the handle. He said, "I think it's killing me". He was right; it was killing him. Roy is one of many who are seized by angina, a distinct pain in the chest caused by a lack of oxygen to the heart. I checked Roy's testosterone levels, which proved what I had already guessed. They were, of  course, subnormal, so I immediately prescribed transdermal testosterone for him. After three months he came in for a check-up and I asked whether or not the vise was still clamping down on his heart. He smiled and replied, "The only vise I know of is in my garage, on my work bench."

It has been shown that testosterone increases the production of nitric oxide, a natural form of nitroglycerine. This drug is prescribed to alleviate chest pains by opening up the coronary arteries. Many studies provide documentation of testosterone's heart healthy effects. Studies dating back to the mid-1970s have shown that men with low levels of testosterone tend to demonstrate high cholesterol and triglyceride levels with low HDL levels. Since then, study after study has proven testosterone reverses all abnormal lipid parameters, protecting us against plaque buildup and heart attacks.

In truth, testosterone affects the heart in so many different ways. It cleans up the heart's passageways (arteries) by lowering LDL. It causes vasodilatation, which allows more blood to the heart, lowering the chance of chest pain. It keeps the HDL at optimal levels. Testosterone and the heart have a long, symbiotic history. When testosterone is at optimal levels, it decreases inflammation in the coronary arteries, thereby reducing heart attacks. Testosterone reduces inflammatory cytokines, which cause plaque rupture and the resulting heart attack and stroke. This well-studied and documented benefit of testosterone is the single most important reason all men should be on optimal testosterone replacement. More than 90 percent of the heart attacks in men could be avoided by preventing endothelial inflammation. This can be accomplished just by maintaining optimal testosterone levels. In light of this outstanding proof, many cardiologists still ignore it as a beneficial therapy. Testosterone lowers fibrinogens, serum triglycerides, total cholesterol, LDL cholesterol and Apo-lipoprotein B, all risk factors of heart disease. Testosterone increases all positive factors and decreases all negative factors.

The Smart Hormone

We spend years experiencing life. For all those good and bad experiences, there is no merit if they cannot be found in the jumbled mess of declining neurons, neurotransmitters, and synapses. The saddest portrait of age is of a person locked away from his or her own mind and memories.

With more and more people living well into their 80s, medicine has to be on its toes to meet the cognitive needs. It is estimated that Alzheimer's disease claims over 4 million people in the United States alone and is the most common cause of dementia. Alzheimer's is recognized by abnormal clumps, referred to as senile plaques and irregular knots called neurofibrillary tangles of brain cells. These two aspects of Alzheimer's disease jumble the memory and the learning processes. A groundbreaking study has revealed testosterone may be a protective accessory to the brain in evading Alzheimer's disease. Researchers are diligently trying to find ways to prevent Alzheimer's disease. It seems hormones are the key that unlocks the door on the mysteries of this debilitating illness.

Since Alzheimer's disease has no cure, the only current therapy is prevention. For the past five years, the New York Academy of Science has presented papers on the powerful effect testosterone has in protecting against the deposition of beta-amyloid protein in the brain, preventing Alzheimer's from occurring. Multiple laboratory studies confirm the protection in lab animals. Many observational studies also confirm reduced incidence with higher levels of testosterone. This is another demonstration that normal testosterone levels are not as protective as optimal levels.

Although testosterone has been adequately demonstrated to protect against Alzheimer's disease, it is felt that the mechanism of action is through conversion of testosterone to estrogen. Many studies have demonstrated estrogen's protective effect against Alzheimer's disease. It's the effect of estrogen on the brain that is the mechanism by which testosterone exerts its protective effects. This is yet another important reason not to block the conversion of testosterone to estrogen or to lower estrogen levels in men.

Month after month, new research pops up and offers the latest word on Alzheimer's disease. Lately, this word seems to be testosterone. These studies, along with others, raise the possibility that Alzheimer's can be stifled at its onset and hormones play a vital role in preventing this disease. Alzheimer's is a disease rarely seen in those under 50. It may not be a coincidence this correlates with the depression of the hormones that sustain us in our youth.

The mind is a powerful and essential part of your being. It mandates how your organs and emotions react to both positive and negative stimuli. The years ahead are worth remembering and testosterone may be the essential tool to keep our brains running like a fine-tuned engine. Many people complain of memory loss. As doctors, we tell them there is nothing we can do to prevent mental deterioration. Nevertheless, as multiple studies demonstrate, hormone replacement is the only method scientifically-proven to protect the brain from dementia, as it also maintains memory function.

Getting the Prostate under Control

Testosterone in association with the prostate has been the subject of much research and much controversy. Contrary to what we are taught, optimal levels of testosterone are the prostate's best resource to health and longevity. Only when testosterone levels decline does the prostate suffer from alterations. Prostate cancer and benign prostatic hypertrophy are age-related diseases. When testosterone is at its highest, prostates are healthy. It is only when age begins to rob the body of testosterone that complications of the prostate arise.

First, I want to discuss the testosterone controversy and testosterone's role in prostate cancer. Androgens have been thought to play a role in the origination and development of prostate disease. This is far from the truth. Androgens do not cause prostate cancer. However, they may cause cell proliferation once the cancer is already present. There is no definitive proof that androgens, specifically testosterone and DHT, initiate cancer in the prostate. A DHT patch is actually in the process of being approved by the FDA. If DHT were so dangerous to the prostate, it is doubtful it would be up for consideration.

Likewise, if testosterone were so dangerous to the prostate gland, it seems that most young men (who have higher testosterone concentrations in the blood) would be suffering from prostate problems. This is not the case. Studies have shown benign prostatic hyperplasia (BPH) and prostate cancers do not correlate with high testosterone levels, nor do PSA levels. BPH and prostate cancer are diseases instigated by age. Since we already know testosterone declines as men get older, it seems to have a valid alibi. Recent studies in the *New England Journal of Medicine* and other peer-viewed medical journals demonstrate testosterone does not cause prostate cancer. Even patients with prostatic intraepithelial neoplasia (early cancer *in situ*), did not go on to develop overt prostate cancer when administered testosterone. There is no medical expert or medical study demonstrating an increased risk of cancer with testosterone administered at optimal levels.

We should be aware of BPH and prostate cancer, but not wary of testosterone therapy. There is a reason men have evaded prostate cancer up until their 40s or 50s. Could this be because testosterone levels have remained where they should be? Optimal testosterone levels are perhaps the best omen for prostatic health. When levels decline, everything is fair game. The prostate seems to be no exception. Every medical study has demonstrated prostate size and symptoms do not increase with testosterone therapy. Many men note improvement in urinary symptoms while on testosterone.

As with breast cancer and estrogen, prostate cancer usually becomes sensitive to testosterone. Even though testosterone does not cause cancer, the tumor may develop receptor sites that become sensitive to testosterone. Treatment may involve blocking testosterone. The presence of prostate cancer certainly precludes use of testosterone to avoid tumor growth. This does not indicate that testosterone provoked the cancer in the first place. However, it may cause it to grow more rapidly if present. It is important to constantly check for prostate cancer by yearly exams and PSA testing. Prostate cancer is the most common cancer in men. Nevertheless, all urology and cancer journals empirically stress that high levels of testosterone or testosterone administration does not increase the risk of prostate cancer.

Although the full discussion is beyond the reach of this book, experts now approve testosterone administration after prostate cancer treatment by surgery or radiation. Once the PSA approaches zero, testosterone can be safely administered. The long-term health benefits of testosterone far outweigh any risks.

What about estrogen and prostate cancer? There has been some data to show estrogen may adversely affect genes which control prostate cancer. However, just as with testosterone, this does not mean estrogen causes prostate cancer. Estrogen produced locally in prostate cells may alter gene expression, but this has nothing to do with serum estrogen levels. Again, 50 years of studies demonstrate that testosterone administration, which raises serum estrogen levels, does not cause prostate cancer.

Estrogen and Progesterone in Men

Although I have briefly addressed this topic earlier in the chapter, this issue is so important and controversial that I must discuss it further. Most physicians know nothing about this subject. The medical literature supports the opposite of what most men are to believe.

Over the last 10 years there has been a growing misconception of estrogen's function in andropause. The neutraceutical industry has fueled the negativism of estrogen as far as prostate function is concerned. Many patients now expect me to measure estrogen levels and prescribe Arimidex® to lower estrogen levels because of the unsubstantiated belief that estrogen is harmful to males. Nothing could be further from the truth. Let me dispel these beliefs and explain why estrogen is so beneficial to males.

Testosterone raises estrogen levels via an enzyme called aromatase. Administering testosterone thereby raises estrogen levels and it is through this aromatase conversion that testosterone exhibits many of its beneficial effects. This is the point that most patients and some physicians do not understand. If estrogen were harmful or problematic, we would have seen it somewhere in the hundreds of studies on testosterone published over the last 40 years. And we don't see any study that demonstrates testosterone increases prostate size, urinary symptoms or prostate cancer, period.

Furthermore there are several studies that demonstrate harm when estrogen is blocked. Men treated with aromatase inhibitors lost bone density, experienced elevated cholesterol levels, and increased heart disease risks. When estrogen was replaced, the cholesterol improved and the bone density improved. We now understand that many of the beneficial effects of testosterone are the direct result of estrogen, which is precisely the reason we do not want to block conversion to estrogen. Estrogen has so many benefits in women and we see those same benefits in men. I can find many studies demonstrating estrogen's beneficial effect in men but I can't find any showing any detriment in all the years that testosterone has been studied.

To take this one step further, it is really the ratio of testosterone that is important and not the level of estrogen. When testosterone is administered, the ratio increases even though the estrogen increases. Correcting the ratio by raising testosterone levels is the important step, not lowering the estrogen. The only time I treat patients with Arimidex® is for increased sensitivity to estrogen that causes breast swelling or tenderness. I will then use Arimidex®, but only to lower estrogen levels slightly to not interfere with the benefits of estrogen. I do not want to lower levels so much that it leads to an increased risk of heart disease, bone loss, Alzheimer's Disease, cholesterol elevation and memory problems. Frequently patients present to me on Arimidex® with estrogen levels at zero. These patients are unaware of the potential harm of suppressing estrogen.

In his book, *The Testosterone Syndrome*, Dr. Eugene Shippen first suggested that estrogen might be harmful. In 2005, Dr. Shippen lectured at a medical conference where he dispelled this myth about estrogen in men. He presented several studies supporting estrogen's beneficial effect in men. Perhaps high levels of estrogen might cause some symptoms in some men, but this does not translate to suppressing estrogen levels at the detriment to one's health. There is no medical evidence that high estrogen levels are harmful, or that low estrogen levels are protective. As above, low estrogen levels have consistently demonstrated increased harm.

Some critics claim that estrogen in men increases the risk of prostate cancer. Yet, this theory is not supported by any medical literature and is purely conjecture. I am not aware of any studies in the last 50 years that have demonstrated an increased risk of prostate cancer is due to elevated estrogen levels. The pharmaceutical literature demonstrates no beneficial effect from aromatase inhibitors (Armidex®) in preventing prostate cancer.

If indeed it did cause it, then we would be blocking estrogen as we do in women. However, this is not the case. In fact, it is the opposite. Several years ago, an alternative prostate cancer treatment became very popular called PC-SPES. This therapy would lower any PSA to below one. Due to manufacturing problems, it was no longer produced and was soon replaced by PC-PLUS, which was even more beneficial in lowering PSA and stopping growth of prostate cancer. The ingredients were Chinese herbs with estrogen-like compounds that were utilized to stop the growth of the prostate and development of cancer. Unfortunately the mechanism of action was to lower testosterone, which causes symptoms associated with low testosterone.

The neutraceutical industry fuels anti-estrogen beliefs by marketing herbal compounds that block conversion (aromatization) of testosterone to estrogen. It is the neutraceutical industry that is to blame for this recent concern over estrogen being harmful in men. Chrysin is one herbal product that is a very weak aromatase inhibitor heavily marketed to consumers. Fortunately it is very weak and hardly blocks aromatization at all. Many patients present to us expecting us to prescribe aromatase inhibitors based on all the literature they read which is primarily from the neutraceutical marketing. These patients are proud to display their knowledge but seem disappointed when we try to convince them otherwise.

Medical science has documented the beneficial effects of testosterone administration. If medical science discovered that blocking the aromatase enzyme was so important, then we would see studies supporting its use and benefits. So far I have not witnessed this in any of my literature reviews. Our research of the literature supports the beneficial effects of estrogen in men. The same research has demonstrated harmful effects when estrogen is lowered. The conclusion therefore is to leave the estrogen alone unless it causes side effects. Research has proven absolutely no harm when prescribed testosterone raises estrogen levels. Perhaps high estrogen and low testosterone levels are harmful, but it is more likely that it is the low testosterone level that is to blame and not the estrogen at all. By raising the testosterone levels, the supposed harm of estrogen disappears. All studies support this and demonstrate there is no harm in raising testosterone or estrogen levels. In contrast, it is more harmful to have deficient, low hormone levels.

Perhaps by now one can appreciate why I preach what I preach. If I recommend or teach a fact, I always support it based on the medical literature. If I cannot adequately support a therapy based on medical literature, then I will not recommend it. On the contrary, if I recommend not using a therapy, this is based on substantial, well-documented scientific studies. I consider myself a messenger who presents the medical literature to support every therapy we recommend, and to condemn therapies not recommended by the medical literature. Documenting and supporting every therapy is truly evidence-based medicine.

On a final note, many practitioners are prescribing progesterone for men based on a false assumption that progesterone protects the prostate. This idea is not demonstrated in any medical literature and is purely hypothetical. Two recent articles demonstrated progesterone's beneficial use in jails, to decrease libido and sexual desire in inmates, which has the same effects of saltpeter (potassium nitrate). Another study demonstrated progesterone had harmful effects on vascular inflammation in men. This inflammation can increase the risk of heart attack and stroke. High levels of progesterone do not exist naturally in men; high levels of estrogen do. Put back in what occurs naturally and this is supported by the medical literature. Progesterone therapy is not medically supported for men, unless you want saltpeter effects and increase in cardiovascular problems. There is significant supposition about raising progesterone levels and lowering estrogen levels in men. I do not understand how it all gets started, but it is pure supposition without any basis in fact. The medical literature provides the evidence that this conjecture is entirely false.

Fine-Tune Yourself for the Years to Come

Remember the story at the beginning of this chapter about the man who had it all? I want to finish the story now.

One of his friends watched patiently as this man presented more and more symptoms all too familiar. He finally decided to intervene and recommended his friend make an appointment to see me. The man found his friend's enthusiasm so irritating he refused to make that appointment for months. In the meantime, his marriage fell into disrepair. His waist size continued to expand even as he doubled his workout time. He found he grew more tired with each passing month. He knew these were the residual signs of getting older, but found no relief in knowing this was a common side effect of aging. He was at an impasse; he felt he was on a one-way street headed for the dead end.

When he finally made his appointment, he grudgingly listened, with his arms folded and facial expression stony. I explained step-by-step what was happening to him. I recounted his downward spiral, verbatim, without his having to tell me anything. I postulated that he felt anxious and depressed. His pants were a little tighter at the waist, he felt sluggish and listless, like the world kept on moving at its same pace while he moved slower and slower. As I concluded, his expression and manner lost its determined disinterest. He had a look of incredulity at my ability to read him like a book.

I assured him that I was no psychic and he was certainly not alone. In fact, he was one of many who visited me each week with the same dilemma. I explained that, if he began a regimen of natural hormone replacement, within months the depression and frustration that had become second nature would dissipate. He would regain his interest in sex and his performance would be optimal. His lean muscle mass would increase and his body fat would decrease. What if he could take something that did all of these things, in addition to boosting heart health, bone density and his overall energy level? Would he do it? His answer was an emphatic "yes." I tested his free testosterone level and put him on an optimal testosterone regimen.

Months after our first visit, I found a renewed man. Life was good, business was great, and he and his wife were going on a second honeymoon. He said the testosterone was life changing, like some miraculous manna.

We take for granted our endocrine system until our hormones sink below their normal levels. It becomes very obvious when the health benefits they once offered fade and the uncomfortable side effects of aging take over. The effects of testosterone supplementation are obvious, and to a deprived man, nothing short of a miracle. The starved receptors receive a sudden jolt of vitality. Men should not go without the essential hormones that once were the spice of their life.

It remains clear: testosterone is a boon to the body. It protects the body against heart disease, osteoporosis, dementia and Alzheimer's. It also revitalizes muscles and skin and significantly enhances the quality of life. In effect, testosterone can transform an ailing man into his healthy mirror image. Age may flip the hormone switch to a lower setting, but now you have the education and the resources to flip the switch back to your more youthful, energetic years. No man should be allowed to suffer the symptoms and consequences of low testosterone.

In Short...

Testosterone's Benefits: Testosterone protects the body against heart disease and osteoporosis and increases a man's sense of well being. It enhances sexual desire and performance and maintains strength and energy. Testosterone enhances muscle tone, strengthens bones, decreases cholesterol levels, and protects the brain against the protein deposits that lead to Alzheimer's disease.

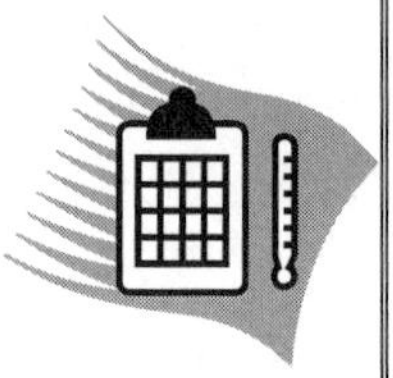

Testosterone's Side Effects: In men with prostate cancer, testosterone may cause the cancer to grow more rapidly; therefore, it should not be administered until PSA levels reach zero, after cancer treatment. Testosterone does not cause the cancer, but may stimulate growth if a cancer does occur.

Bottom Line: Raising a man's testosterone to optimal levels through natural hormone replacement therapy helps men to regain the positive, healthy aspects of their younger years in every aspect of their lives.

Testosterone: The Woman's Side of the Story

Testosterone completely shot up my libido. It seemed I wanted sex just as I did when I was twenty.

—Felicia, 43

I heard that testosterone caused abnormal hair growth. When my doctor prescribed it, all I could imagine is what I would look like with a beard in a new job as a sideshow act. Boy, was I wrong. I feel like a butterfly hatched from a long cocooned sleep. I feel sexy and colorful—a far cry from the circus act I imagined. My energy, appearance, and attitude have totally changed.

—Kharen, 56

Many women find it surprising that testosterone is produced in the ovary along with estrogen and progesterone, just as men are shocked by the idea that their bodies thrive with the help of estrogen. Women are also stunned by the news that testosterone is vital for good female health, including bone growth and sex drive.

Testosterone levels in the female body are about 10 percent of the amount found in men. This 10 percent makes all the difference. Testosterone has been found to enhance sex drive and mood, while working to maintain bone health and lean muscle mass. Testosterone is as essential to a female's health and well being as progesterone and estrogen. Unfortunately, testosterone has been left off the female hormone roster. This exclusion leaves a woman incomplete.

There seems to be an irrational fear pervading our society pertaining to women and testosterone.

Some people believe women undergo a masculine transformation, when they are administered testosterone. Hair will grow on the face, the voice will deepen, and the personality will take on a more masculine temperament. I'm here to tell you this is a silly paranoia brought on by lack of experience, understanding, and overactive imaginations. Nevertheless, you wouldn't believe the aversion displayed by some of my female patients when I prescribe them what has been falsely proclaimed as the "male" hormone. However, once they have been on testosterone for a few months, they're singing quite a different tune. Of all the hormones we replace, testosterone is responsible for most of the feel-good effects from hormone replacement therapy.

Adverse side effects only occur at high, irresponsible dosages and usually only with synthetic hormones. A trained physician will tailor each hormone program around the specific needs of their patient. I use blood levels as well as a woman's symptoms to calculate dosages that will effectively and safely raise levels up into more youthful ranges. After six weeks of initial therapy, each patient has a follow-up appointment. I recheck her levels and make the necessary dosage adjustments. Studies that convey concerns about women taking testosterone could have seen ill effects if dosages were too high. Tragically, these studies received a large amount of press. Other studies, dating back to the late 1950s, claiming that testosterone enhanced sexuality and energy, were buried and forgotten. Recent articles appearing in the *Journal of the American Medical Association* and *New England*

Journal of Medicine have demonstrated there are no side effects from testosterone in these large studies.

Not just laymen confuse testosterone replacement in women as something unneeded and dangerous; doctors too, have often perpetuated this myth. This is why only a very small percentage of women are getting the full and complete benefit from their hormone regimen. Without testosterone, women get the main course without the spice that makes it interesting and palatable. I'm writing this chapter separately from the main testosterone chapter as I feel women suffer their own testosterone deficiency. On top of menopause, they also suffer a form of andropause. Although women receive prescriptions for estrogen and progesterone, they have to battle social fashion and unfounded fears to supplement testosterone. Testosterone must be replaced just as estrogen and progesterone. Unfortunately many physicians and patients are unfamiliar and unaware of the tremendous benefits of testosterone. Women who read Suzanne Somers' book *The Sexy Years*, will arrive at their doctor's office begging for testosterone.

Women need to rise above rumors instigated even more by inertia than ignorance. They should enjoy the full spectrum of hormone replacement therapy. Women must also realize that the side effects mentioned are from old studies that utilized synthetic testosterone. Recent studies on bio identical testosterone now report minimal side effects.

Are You in the Mood?

Let's Get Technical: Testosterone Production in Women

Testosterone is formed in both the ovaries and the adrenal glands. It travels through the body via the blood, but most is attached to the protein, sex hormone-binding globulin. Only 1 to 3 percent of testosterone is free to link up with tissues and produce the desired hormonal response. Even in that small amount, there is a time-related drop in testosterone 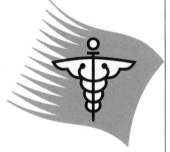 beginning after a woman is in her 20s. This decrease continues as a woman passes through menopause and her ovaries become dormant and her adrenal glands slow down.

Testosterone production decreases as does the adrenal glands' production of DHEA and androstendione. When these declines take place, a woman feels a stark absence in sexual arousal. Basically, testosterone is the stuff desire is made of. Just as testosterone flips a switch in boys during puberty, testosterone also aids girls in their sexual awakening. It is testosterone that stimulates the growth of pubic and underarm hair. It has specific receptors located in the breasts, vagina, and clitoris. Testosterone's presence stimulates the sensations that women feel in sexual situations. It's basically the tool that turns a woman on.

When testosterone levels drop and sexual desire dissipates, women find they are trapped in a medical world unwilling to help. They are up against conventional wisdom which defines their lack of sexual desire as a mental block, rather than a block in their testosterone production. I have encountered many a female patient frustrated and humiliated by the medical care they have received. These patients don't understand how this "neurosis" developed only after they entered the perimenopause, menopause or postmenopause process.

Read more!

Dr. Susan Rako, in her book *The Hormone of Desire: The Truth About Sexuality, Menopause and Testosterone*, couldn't have said it better: "Menopause is a journey through poorly-charted waters and most physicians approach the possibility of prescribing supplementary testosterone for women suffering symptoms of its deficiency with the resistance and ignorance of sailors who believed the earth was flat, and that if they proceeded to sail on, they would fall off."

This chapter is specifically for women butting their heads against traditional medicine. Your sudden sexual dysfunction is not a mental problem, nor does it lie in uncharted waters. There is research confirming testosterone supplementation helps sexual apathy as well as aiding in a number of other facets influencing sexual appetite, like mood and energy. I want to supply every woman with enough clinical ammunition to challenge any doctor who tells them there is no correlation between lack of sexual desire and low testosterone levels. Pull this book out and point to the sources that say differently.

In women, testosterone levels actually fall over time. Levels peak while women are in their 20s and slowly decrease with each passing year. Once a woman hits menopause, testosterone is usually at an all-time low. This drop is magnified by symptoms of estrogen and progesterone deficiencies.

The most obvious effect of testosterone depletion is the lack of sexual desire. One of my female patients described this as a deadening. "I just feel like that part of my life is over. I've tried everything from the Kama Sutra to just plain smut and nothing seems to awaken my comatose sexual desire." After supplementing testosterone for a few months she smiled shyly at her follow up appointment. When I asked her about her sex life, "Let's just say a miracle has occurred - it has been resurrected."

Women experience a gradual sexual decline as they age. Coupled with the onset of menopause, women experience an even lower rate of coital frequency. Estrogen replacement helps to a certain degree by decreasing bothersome menopausal symptoms. Estrogen is most effective in increasing vaginal moisture. Libido is the primary responsibility of testosterone. Study after study confirms midlife sexual dysfunction is easily eliminated with testosterone supplementation. With testosterone supplementation, women experience not only a sexual surge, but a jump start which throws their sex life into full throttle. Women may begin to experience a resurgence of visual fantasies and multiple orgasms as testosterone levels are optimized. All studies demonstrate an increase in sexual pleasure, frequency, fantasies and intensity and quantity of orgasms. There are many other reasons to supplement testosterone, not just for sex.

Several studies have compared sexual parameters as they relate to estrogen therapy alone or estrogen replacement coupled with testosterone therapy. All studies seem to agree estrogen alone has no influence on a woman's sexual health. When combined with testosterone, the changes women experience are amazing both in attitude and ability. The two sex hormones work hand in hand to create a healthy physical and emotional environment.

One study is particularly interesting. It implies estrogen replacement may be somewhat of an inhibitor to the testosterone a woman creates after menopause. I'm not saying women should stop estrogen because it boosts the production of SHBG. Estrogen provides far too many valuable resources for the heart, bones and vagina. Testosterone curbs estrogen's influence on the overproduction of SHBG. What I do suggest is that women supplement testosterone along with their other hormones. This way, supplemental testosterone is more available to remain free and active for bodily tissues, while estrogen is able to benefit the heart, bones and mind.

While many women are on estrogen replacement alone, there are some who receive the added benefits of natural progesterone. A very small number receive the advantages of testosterone replacement. So many women are led to believe sexual listlessness resides in their head, a blatant psychological setback. Unfortunately, they are misdiagnosed and treated improperly. For many of these women, this therapy is frustrating and embarrassing. A good indicator for testosterone deficiency is a loss of sexual responsiveness in all phases, not only sexual arousal but sexual desire. Many women are prescribed antidepressants, which further lower libido and sexual response.

I had a patient whom we'll call Linda. She felt guilty over her lack of response to her husband's advances. She hadn't always felt that way, and this new negativity toward intimacy created a rift in their marriage. She went to counseling for several months and later described it to me as "therapy that entailed hitting her head against the wall"— it offered no clue to her sexual inhibition.

I measured her total and free testosterone levels and discovered they were quite low. After the proper dosage and several months later, Linda called to say she was no longer banging her head against the wall and her husband thanks me for it.

Testosterone replacement can reawaken a patient's optimism and energy. I believe vitality and enhanced mood alone can boost a woman's sex drive. Any woman overwhelmed by fatigue and depression is challenged to feel sexual desire. I am positive that an increase in energy and optimism quickly leads to sexual contentment. Several tests have indicated that testosterone bolsters optimism and vigor in surgically menopausal women.

This segment is for all women whose sexual comfort has been ignored. Testosterone is a potent remedy for sexual dysfunction. It is time to ask your doctor to measure your testosterone levels. If he or she is opposed, find a doctor who will. With prudent judgment and proper monitoring, you can regain your sexuality and feel content in your life.

Age does not mean abstinence, and it certainly does not mean displeasure. Intimacy is as necessary to health as a proper diet. If you are one of the many women out there experiencing a sexual slump, snap out of it and have your testosterone levels checked. You could experience your own sexual reawakening. I treat a number of women over 80 who are open and honest about their sex lives. The quantity and quality they experience would make a younger woman jealous.

Building Bone with Hormones

Most people have been taught to consume calcium by drinking glasses of milk each day. We know vitamin D somehow affects the bone. What a lot of people don't know is that our sex hormones play a substantial role in the delicate balance of bone reproduction. You can drink glass after glass of milk and pop vitamin D all you want, but as we get older, our hormones will decline; our bones will become weaker.

How many times have you seen an older person warped by age? It's a sobering portrait of a body without the proper defenses to ward off aging. Doctors and researchers have observed how our bones survive over the years by constant reconstruction. Our bones are dynamic works of art that need maintenance for a proper equilibrium.

We have a construction crew of specialized cells, called osteoblasts and osteoclasts, which work with one another to either build or tear down bone. When our hormones decline, the equilibrium between these cells breaks down, and osteoclasts run amuck, reabsorbing more bone than is being made. The relationship between bone loss and aging is not a coincidence. It is not a twist of fate that when hormones are added back to the female body, there is a remarkable increase in bone density.

Research now shows that when testosterone is incorporated into a woman's hormone treatment program, there is an improvement in bone density. This improvement is more dramatic than estrogen and progesterone supplementation alone. Doctors are finding that levels of bio-available testosterone are predictors, in men and women, of height loss and subsequent vertebral fractures. Other studies have shown that small amounts of testosterone added to estrogen increased bone formation by 50 percent over a three-month period. By including just a small amount of testosterone in your hormone replacement program, you could potentially improve your bone loss by up to 41 percent. These percentages alone should be enough to make you call your doctor for an appointment. Testosterone has been shown to be much better for bone growth than estrogen, calcium and vitamin D.

The estrogen/testosterone combination has proven to be osteoporosis's formidable enemy. The recipe for bone health has been missing an important ingredient in most HRT programs. Testosterone has been overlooked or pushed aside as something unessential to the female body. I find this amusing, since a woman has been manufacturing testosterone on her own for many years and the body never does anything without a purpose. Testosterone is a bonus for bone health, but unfortunately many women never get the extra boost.

I'm surprised when women come to my office on synthetic hormones and have never heard of natural hormones. Their vitality has plunged and their sex life is nonexistent. Worse still, their bones are wasting away. It is the right of every woman to request all essential hormones in a bio identical compound.

More Side Benefits of Testosterone for Women

Many times, when people discuss hormone replacement therapy, they focus on the side effects. Yet, when a woman's testosterone is restored to optimal levels, she will experience what I call "side benefits." One of the most pleasant of the "side benefits" is the revitalization of skin texture. Testosterone increases collagen content and elasticity in the skin to prevent wrinkles. Another "side benefit" is the ability to attain the youthful shape you once had. Testosterone adds muscle back to the body which supports the curves you once had. Your fat to muscle ratio flips, and you'll notice a more toned and defined figure. You will quickly discover you have more energy and the desire to be more active. Your strength and endurance will surprise you. You won't fatigue as easily and your joints won't ache like they used to.

Dr. Don Gambrell, Jr., a clinical professor of endocrinology, obstetrics, and gynecology encourages adding a low-dose androgen to the estrogen replacement regimen. He wrote that the potential benefits include the lessening of:

- Hot flashes
- Lethargy
- Endogenous depression
- Nocturia and incontinence
- Fibrocystic disease of the breast
- Vascular headaches
- Poor libido

> **Let's Get Technical: Cardiovascular Protection**
> Studies have shown testosterone also has cardiovascular protective functions. A combination of testosterone and estrogen has been shown to have beneficial effects on the cardiovascular system, especially concerning lipids, atherogenesis, and vasodilation. It has been shown to improve good cholesterol and lower triglyceride levels.

Testosterone, like progesterone, is absolutely necessary to add to your estrogen replacement regimen. With the combination of all three hormones, a woman can feel like herself again. She will experience a reawakening, not only in her spirits, but also her skin and the shape of her body. We usually refer to young women as being in full bloom. I have seen many women on a complete hormone replacement program of testosterone, estrogen, and progesterone literally bloom like a perennial blossom.

I urge you to discover the nourishing qualities these essential hormones have on the outside and inside of your body. They are the fuel on which your vital organs and tissues thrive. Hormones are truly what allow you to grow young and healthy through the years.

Testosterone: The Female Hormone

Testosterone as the "male hormone" is a misnomer. Testosterone is just as much a female hormone. If anyone tells you differently, they have not studied their general human biology. Society as a whole feels safer when things are in compartments: estrogen is a female hormone; testosterone is a male hormone, thus the uproar and obstinacy over testosterone supplementation in women.

The human body is complex. It is now time to break free of the constrictions of simple thinking. Testosterone is a female hormone and your health deserves first-rate care. Female sexuality, in particular, needs specific attention. We've seen the token portraits of a "dried-up" middle-aged woman who has become stingy with her sexuality. It is not stinginess, only a middle-aged testosterone deficiency. This is not as good as it gets. Fortunately you have many great years ahead. Take charge and incorporate a natural hormone program into your life. Spice it up with just the right ingredient. You have the curiosity—that's why you're reading this book. Now you need a nudge. Well, here it is:

Testosterone is like fertilizer. In the years that I've been taking it, I feel taller and brighter and fresher than I have in a long time.

—Judy, age 55

I never thought I would say this again...but I love sex!

—Mary, age 59

...and the energy, I actually thought my doctor laced my cream with some sort of illegal stimulant. I never thought I would feel this good.

—Isabel, age 61

In Short...

Testosterone's benefits: Testosterone can produce improvement in well being, energy, body composition, bone density, sexual function, and clitoral sensitivity. Testosterone has many health benefits in preventing skin wrinkles and skin thinning from loss of collagen. Testosterone protects against deterioration of muscle, ligaments, joint, tendons, bone and skin – anything that has to do with our structure and aesthetics.

Testosterone's side effects: Doses that are irresponsibly large can cause abnormal hair growth and acne. In low doses, there are no serious side effects.

The Bottom Line: Testosterone isn't just for men. It can make all the difference in women living a vibrant life as they age. Testosterone is the feel-good hormone for both men and women.

Thyroid:
The Most Misunderstood Hormone

*After turning 40, I started noticing a progressive
increase in fatigue. When others were warm, I was cold.
My periods became irregular and my bowels became
constipated. I felt drained of energy and drive. I gained 15
pounds. I went to several doctors, who either prescribed me
some form of antidepressant or brushed me off as being a
hypochondriac. I felt worse on the antidepressants and I was
frustrated with the lack of help or sympathy I was
receiving from my health care providers.*
—Lisa, 45

I have encountered so many people who say they are
truly unhealthy and unhappy—even after seeing every kind of
doctor from endocrinologists to acupuncturists. People still
have complaint after complaint. Although their hormone
levels seem normal, their doctors just can't pinpoint exactly
what ails them. They are positive they are not in good health.
When in actuality they are somewhat healthy—except for one
small but significant problem. These people suffer from
thyroid insufficiency—a very common problem that is
overlooked by many physicians.

When Lisa was referred to me, she viewed me with a
skepticism she had developed from her previous health-care
experiences.

Her story was not unusual to me and she seemed baffled
at my curiosity and probing questions. I measured her TSH
(thyroid-stimulating hormone) level, along with her free T3
and T4 levels. She was definitely suffering from an
insufficiency in thyroid, although this was the first time
anyone had mentioned her thyroid. Many doctors measured

her TSH levels (I'll explain what that is later), along with other standard tests, and found that her levels were "normal."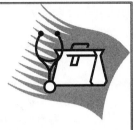

In spite of her normal levels, I treated her anyway with a natural thyroid hormone. She had become resigned to thinking her problem was "in her mind," and was relieved to find out that it was her Free T-3 levels that were out of whack and not her head after all.

After three weeks, she felt better. "I can actually wake up in the morning and look forward to seeing my husband and going to work. I don't crash or have to nap halfway through the day."

After two months, her added pounds began to fall off. At her follow-up appointment, the dark circles under her eyes disappeared, and she smiled. "I'm going shopping after our visit to celebrate how good I look and feel."

Many doctors feel more inclined to treat blood levels rather than symptoms. This philosophy results in treating the lab test and not the person, a philosophy that makes healthcare very frustrating. As is in most cases, the lab tests are normal to low normal and the patient is just written off. Despite the normal test results, the symptoms people experience will only be resolved when they are treated with thyroid hormone replacement. Remember, normal does not equate to optimal.

More often than not, patient's labs are misread or perhaps their symptoms are merely overlooked. This allows for hypothyroidism (under-active thyroid) to go unchecked and untreated. Unfortunately, unchecked or untreated hypothyroidism will only worsen over time.

There are three different types of low thyroid conditions. The first type, primary hypothyroidism, is easy to diagnose. However, most patients suffer from the second or third type.

In Dr. Gerald S. Levey's article, *"Hypothyroidism: A Treacherous Masquerader,"* he refers to the illness as a subtle illness that eludes doctors. The illness is accompanied by a melting pot of symptoms. Often, thyroid insufficiency or hypothyroidism is misconstrued in people older than 50 or 60 as normal symptoms of aging. Fatigue, slower speech, forgetfulness, weight gain, depression, hair loss, and the tendency to feel cold are all symptoms normally associated with aging. However, they are more related to the symptoms of an aging thyroid. The traditional medical community will usually try to treat these symptoms in younger patients, but feel it unnecessary to do the same for older patients.

If you feel age has crept up and you recognize the above symptoms, please do not accept this as simply the facts of life. You should not have to tolerate these symptoms as they can be successfully treated.

As women age, they are more likely than men to experience hypothyroid symptoms. The problem here is symptoms of hypothyroidism often overlap with those of perimenopause and menopause. Although a woman may be receiving estrogen and progesterone to eliminate her menopausal symptoms, many symptoms persist due to thyroid insufficiency.

I remember a patient, a teacher, whose estrogen and progesterone levels were restored to normal, yet she couldn't shake her depression and fatigue.

"I couldn't focus on my lessons. I had a hard time being creative with my students and my attention span was poor. I couldn't capture the interest of my students. All I wanted to do was stay in bed. I had no idea how significant the thyroid was until I started taking it. What a relief to find a doctor who understood the problem and could successfully treat it."

It took her several doctors and several unsuccessful antidepressants to finally get referred to me. Her symptoms were so classic—hair falling out, brittle fingernails, coarse skin, and lethargy; I was surprised no one had thought to check her thyroid, let alone treat it.

When a woman suffers from hypothyroidism, it deeply affects the menopausal process. Since the symptoms are similar (i.e. forgetfulness, depression, mood swings, muscle weakness, change in skin or hair texture, sleep disturbances, anxiety or irritability, palpitations and irregular periods), many doctors overlook the thyroid and prescribe the normal menopausal treatment. For many women, this does the trick in eliminating the bothersome menopausal symptoms. But for those women who cannot shake depression and fatigue even after estrogen and progesterone supplementation, they need to have their thyroid levels checked. More often than not, they will find their levels are "low-normal" or insufficient. If their levels are low-normal, the doctor may brush over them without notice as they still fall in the "normal" range. However, the levels need to be restored to optimal ranges if a persons wishes to enjoy a healthy and happy life again.

This is exactly where the misunderstanding and confusion lie. Most people over the age of 40 have low-normal baseline levels. Normal is not optimal. Normal can cause a person to experience multiple symptoms of hypothyroidism. Many patients will not improve until their thyroid levels are supplemented into the upper range of normal. When thyroid levels are raised to the upper range, symptoms resolve, health improves, and patients truly feel the difference. According to the medical literature, optimal levels are needed to reap the benefits of thyroid. "Normal" means you are just as low as everyone else your age.

Thyroid is an Essential Hormone

Like all essential hormones, thyroid levels decrease as we age. Thyroid insufficiency or hypothyroidism commonly occurs. Insufficiencies often go undetected. This problem is even more widespread than typically reported. One of the interesting things about thyroid supplementation is most patients experience significant improvement and feel much better once their serum levels are optimized. Symptomatic improvement occurs when serum levels reach this optimal range. Serum levels in the low-normal to mid-normal range are not where a person feels good.

Every hormone our body produces is necessary for good health. Thyroid is one of the most vital hormones as it affects every organ, cell, and hormone in the body. The body cannot survive without its presence. When thyroid is simply deficient, the body can suffer from high cholesterol and triglyceride levels, sluggish thought process, memory impairment, weight gain, cold intolerance, constipation, menstrual abnormalities and changes in hair, skin, and nails.

It can be difficult to identify thyroid as the culprit given the vastness of the symptomatic spectrum. Many times, patients are shuffled from one doctor to the next and one medication to the other. Low thyroid-induced depression may be treated with an anti-depressant. Hypothyroid-influenced weight gain may be attributed to a poor diet and exercise regimen. When a person is suffering from hypothyroidism or insufficient thyroid levels, an anti-depressant or a low-fat diet/high-caliber exercise program is a waste of time. In spite of normal thyroid levels on a standard blood test, improvement is only accomplished when thyroid is replenished to optimal levels.

Along with the thyroid enigma, controversy surrounds the type of thyroid medication which should be used for treatment. Some doctors believe the synthetic form (Synthroid®, Levoxyl®, T4) works the best. Other doctors support the natural, desiccated thyroid. I sit firmly in the Rouzier camp, natural is best. Later in this chapter, I will present the details of the debate and the differences between the two types of hormones. You will quickly understand my position on natural thyroid and why many of my forward-thinking colleagues have joined me in prescribing natural thyroid.

Natural thyroid most effectively raises the active thyroid hormone called T3. Natural thyroid contains a combination of T4 and T3 and will provide more optimal results than Synthroid® and other synthetic T4 preparations. Since T3 is the more metabolic hormone, low T3 levels result in poor metabolism and thyroid insufficiencies. When pure T4 is given in the form of Synthroid® or Levoxyl®, T3 levels only minimally improve. Many physicians, including endocrinologists, believe T4 is the thyroid preparation to prescribe. The reasoning behind their belief is that the body will automatically convert T4 to T3. This belief is based on theory and not on data. Recent studies show T4 does not adequately convert to T3. Adding T3 to the T4 preparation allows us to optimize T3 levels. This was recently published in the *New England Journal of Medicine*.

Potential thyroid problems include:
1) Lack of production of thyroid hormone.
2) Lack of conversion of T4 to T3, which causes low T3 levels and symptoms of low thyroid.
3) Typically prescribed T4 preparations that do not adequately convert to T3, which causes symptoms of low thyroid even adequate amounts of T4 are supplemented.
4) Receptor site insensitivity in spite of adequate thyroid levels results in low thyroid symptoms.

Your Amazing Thyroid

Your thyroid is the butterfly shaped gland that wraps around the front of your windpipe. It varies in weight, but is usually about one ounce. Fascinatingly enough, the thyroid gland only secretes a tablespoon of this metabolic hormone a year. The

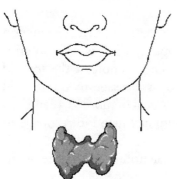

majority of it is bound to a protein, making it useless to tissues. This seemingly insignificant amount makes a world of difference to your body. Thyroid:

- Is critical to the growth, differentiation, and metabolism of each cell in the body.
- Regulates temperature,

metabolism, and cerebral function.

- Increases breakdown of fat and lowers cholesterol levels, protecting you against heart disease.
- Increases your cerebral metabolism and prevents cognitive decline.

Let's Get Technical: Thyroid Hormones

Thyroid hormones help regulate our growth and metabolism. They also help to set our sleep rhythms. The two most important hormones that the thyroid secretes are:

- Thyroxine, also known as T4
- Triiodothyronine, known as T3

About 80 percent of the thyroid hormone we produce is T4, the weaker thyroid hormone. T3, the active hormone, makes up only about 20 percent of the thyroid hormone, yet is four times stronger than T4. Most of the thyroid's metabolic effect is due to T3 and not T4. It is the conversion of T4 to T3 that makes the thyroid active. T4 is therefore more of a pro-hormone or hormone precursor to the more active thyroid hormone called T3.

Another important hormone involved in thyroid function is TSH (also known as thyrotropin). TSH is the anterior pituitary hormone that stimulates the function of the thyroid gland. It is the hormone that sends a message to the thyroid gland in the neck and tells it to make more T4 and T3 hormones. It is produced by the pituitary gland in response to signals from the hypothalamus gland.

The thyroid also produces calcitonin which helps us metabolize calcium and strengthens our bones.

Thyroid dysfunction can occur as an age-related insensitivity to the receptor sites. Traditional medicine often resists this idea that receptor sites become desensitized with age. Yet, there are times when patients have all the symptoms of hypothyroidism and the outcome of all their thyroid tests are normal. These patients are usually left to fend for themselves because the numbers do not reflect a thyroid insufficiency. Unfortunately, many doctors opt to treat the numbers, rather than the symptoms. For these patients, if thyroid hormone is prescribed, the symptoms seldom resolve, giving credence to thyroid resistance or the receptor insensitivity theory.

As we age, thyroid resistance and receptor insensitivity are actually the most common cause of low thyroid symptoms. This is most frustrating for patients as they wander from doctor to doctor only to find their thyroid tests are normal. Fortunately, their symptoms improve when they find a physician willing to treat their symptoms and prescribe natural thyroid hormones.

Many doctors never equate low free T3 levels with the signature symptoms of thyroid insufficiency. If TSH and T4 levels are normal, most physicians will end their examination of thyroid function. It is now your responsibility to educate yourself on thyroid options and present them to your doctor. If your doctor remains unreceptive, search for a new doctor who will listen. It is your body, and perhaps you are the most aware of exactly what it needs and exactly what it can do without.

Why am I Always Cold?

Are you cold to the touch? Are your hands like an ice cube? Do your feet never get warm? Are you always freezing at work when your co-workers find the temperature just right? You are not alone. Many people are faced with these same complaints. They are actually one of the tell-tale signs of thyroid insufficiency.

One of my patients -- we'll call her Deana -- had lived for several years feeling, as she put it, "chilled to the bone." Many patients with thyroid insufficiency will constantly complain of cold hands and cold feet.

She had been to her general practitioner, who had checked her TSH level and found it to be normal. Instead of treating the symptoms, he simply treated the blood test and sent her on her way.

When she came to see me with another problem, she mentioned how cold she felt all the time. "I live in Southern California, and I feel as if I'm at the North Pole. I'm freezing." Deana was also tired quite often and fell into unexplainable lows throughout the day. She frequently felt drained of energy. "Even if I get a good solid eight hours of sleep, I still can't keep my eyes open."

She was surprised at my interest in her story, as she was used to this abnormality as a fact of life. We tested her free T3 levels and found that she was abnormally low and certainly not optimal.

After a month of thyroid supplementation her thyroid levels went back to optimal. Deana had a stable level of energy throughout the day and she didn't have to wear a sweater to work anymore.

She called to say, "So this is what Southern California feels like." She was so pleased with the improvement of her thin skin, hair, and nails. Although many women complain of thin hair, skin and nails, these symptoms, often wrongly attributed to aging, are only reversed by adequate and optimal thyroid supplementation.

After years of shaking hands with low-thyroid patients, I have become adept at guessing their thyroid function by simply shaking their hands. The colder the hands, the lower the thyroid function.

Optimal thyroid levels govern the metabolic process, which is what determines how hot or cold you feel. If your temperature dips below normal, the pituitary gland increases TSH production, which in turn, provokes a production of thyroid. In this way, the body generates the heat to offset cold temperatures. When thyroid levels dip, so does the body's temperature. However, for many women, the TSH does not change and they are left feeling uncomfortably cold. This is due to either low T3 levels or decreased sensitivity to thyroid hormone. The treatment is the same: raising T3 to optimal levels, which reverses the symptoms.

At optimal levels, the thyroid regulates the body's temperature, which manages important processes like the workings of the immune system and cerebral function. When our bodies are at the right temperature, 98.6 degrees, they are able to work efficiently. Normal temperatures are essential for proper enzyme function and preservation of health.

Although the thyroid affects temperature and warmth, not every patient with low thyroid function will experience cold symptoms. There are more than 200 symptoms related to low thyroid functions and many patients experience only one to two of the symptoms. Some people may experience very mild symptoms, while others experience very severe symptoms.

News to Cure the Blues

Depression and fatigue top the list of the most common symptoms of insufficient thyroid levels. For various reasons, these symptoms often go misdiagnosed or ignored. Doctors blame mood swings and weariness on the stress of life. They perform basic blood tests, which includes measuring the TSH, finding no problems there. From here, doctors start prescribing different medications: anti-anxiety, anti-depressants, sleep aids, only to finally refer patients to psychiatrists.

Think of the dismay when patients realize their arsenal of medications only make them feel worse. They didn't have the proper blood tests so there was no indication they were suffering from low T3 levels and thyroid insufficiency.

Women, more often than men, find themselves trapped and feel ignored. Unfortunately, many of them suffer for a long time before they find a doctor who listens to the symptoms, orders the proper tests, and considers both when making a diagnosis and treatment plan.

When it comes to something as elusive as hypothyroidism or low-normal thyroid levels, traditional medical doctors rely exclusively on blood tests. If the blood tests reveal no abnormality, they declare the patient healthy. They often dismiss the symptoms as psychosomatic, and prescribe antidepressants.

Diagnostic tests should be looked upon as a guide that allows the doctor to more thoroughly understand and treat the patient. If a doctor will listen to the symptoms presented by the patient, and treat the patient rather than the test, they will find the results amazing. My dictum is that any depression, fatigue or "feeling lousy" are due to thyroid deficiency unless proven otherwise.

Mary Shoman, a long-time researcher on thyroid insufficiency, administered a poll at a thyroid forum. She asked people what they felt were the worst symptoms of thyroid disease. More than 700 people answered the poll. Twenty three percent believed their depression problems were directly related and were the most difficult problem to deal with.

The thyroid not only plays a critical role in our physical well-being, but also affects our emotional well being. When the thyroid is at proper levels, stressful events are handled with ease, and fatigue is not a common, unexplainable occurrence. If thyroid levels dip, fatigue, depression, mood swings, and mental sluggishness can seriously hamper a patient's physical and emotional well-being.

Psychiatrists often describe depression as a "chemical deficiency in the brain." Loss of the brain hormone serotonin results in depression. However, loss of thyroid hormone can affect the brain in a similar way. Because the thyroid regulates metabolism and influences most major organs in your body, it is no wonder many thyroid patients feel unhappy and fatigued when their levels are not optimal.

Low thyroid levels have such widespread effects, as a person's self-esteem and self-perception are often affected. Skin and hair become dry, nails get brittle, pounds accumulate, the patient feels tired and "on the edge." This all adds up to depression. The patient's body is essentially reacting to the absence of thyroid.

Even when a patient's hypothyroidism or low thyroid levels have been detected, he or she is often prescribed the wrong kind of thyroid to adequately correct the deficiency. This commonly results in the persistence of symptoms despite treatment.

One of my patients, "Janet," had been diagnosed with hypothyroidism and treated with Synthroid® over a year's span.

Although her hypothyroidism had been treated, Janet still had persistent symptoms of low thyroid function.

A friend suggested that she come to me. I listened to her story and let her know that she was on the wrong thyroid medication. I showed her an article from the *New England Journal of Medicine* that explained how many times patients have more success and feel better faster if they used a natural thyroid preparation that raises T3 levels much better than T4. I gave her a prescription for natural thyroid and asked her to call me in a few weeks.

When she called, she had nothing but positive things to say. "It's amazing," she said. She was frustrated only that it took so long to diagnose and treat the problem.

A lack of sufficient thyroid levels can also make it nearly impossible for a patient to think clearly. Patients complain their fatigue is clouding their minds. This cognitive haze is not uncommon.

Many doctors lack confidence in supplementing thyroid without supporting blood results. You may think this is overstated. Well, I promise you it is not. In fact, it cannot be stated enough. Many physicians lack the understanding and experience necessary to supplement thyroid hormone when the lab tests are normal. Physicians must be trained in this regard and have the knowledge and ability to optimize thyroid function by prescribing natural thyroid hormone (T3 and T4). The responsibility of a doctor should be to increase the well being of his or her patients despite the lab tests. Remember, treat the patient not the number. Contemporary studies in some of our best medical journals are coming around to the same conclusions.

I find it amazing that patients with symptoms of depression are rarely checked for thyroid dysfunction. I find it even more amazing that if hypothyroidism is detected, they are given a hormone supplement that will not supply them with adequate thyroid levels. Therefore, their symptomatic depression symptoms rarely subside.

Study after study has proven that patients will feel better on optimal thyroid therapy, even if their TSH initially tested normal. Physicians should focus on the free T3 level and raise it to optimal levels. Only then will symptoms subside. A recent study from the *Journal of Clinical Endocrine Metabolism*, concluded patients felt the best on the highest amount of T3, which causes TSH suppression.

Weak from Fatigue?

In Mary Shoman's survey, hypothyroid sufferers cited fatigue and exhaustion as their number one problematic symptom (34 percent of respondents). You get a good night's rest, but your days are filled with a vexing sluggishness. When your metabolic rate slows down, you slow down.

Doctors across America record more than 500 million patient visits in regards to fatigue and the sad thing is patients rarely find a cure. Being tired has become as familiar to them as breathing. The complaint of fatigue is baffling to many doctors. They sidestep the cause by recommending exercise programs, healthy diets, and more sleep. All good advice, yet the patient is no closer to discovering the root of the problem and no closer to finding a cure. If a person is hypothyroid or simply suffering from low levels of thyroid, I can promise, a healthy diet and exercise program paired with eight hours of sleep will not eliminate the exhaustion.

Studies have shown, as have my own observation of my patients, that the supplementation of a natural thyroid T4/T3 combination will eliminate a patient's troubling fatigue. Fatigue is not a normal part of one's hectic life, nor is it a typical aspect of growing old.

The cure is easy. Finding a doctor willing to prescribe the cure is the hard part. Once you are on the right type of thyroid, at the correct dose, you will notice a world of difference. You will feel much better and reclaim your active lifestyle.

Thyroid for the Heart?

The heart can also suffer the consequences of thyroid dysfunction. The heart and the thyroid gland are inseparable. Both play a critical role in a person's longevity. How does the thyroid fit into the heart-healthy equation? When functioning well, the thyroid helps to keep blood pressure and cholesterol low and to prevent excessive weight gain. All of these factors are important for heart health. Optimal thyroid levels also regulate a person's metabolism and energy level, two more factors critical in maintaining a healthy heart.

One of the big problems with thyroid insufficiency is that many times patients do not experience the physical and obvious symptoms of hypothyroidism. Their lives are not always afflicted by depression, intolerance to cold, low metabolism, dry skin, or mental and physical lethargy. However, their hearts still suffer from this altered thyroid status. They have an increase in cholesterol and blood pressure, along with hardened arteries.

The Rotterdam Study focused on the effects of sub clinical hypothyroidism (thyroid insufficiency). Researchers were able to show that women with sub-clinical hypothyroidism were more likely to have a history of heart attacks and heart disease. These women had twice the chance of developing atherosclerosis or a heart attack. This and other studies demonstrate that the lower the level of thyroid, the higher the risk for heart disease.

The Rotterdam Study is important to understand, since many times thyroid testing takes place only when symptoms appear. Sometimes, with low normal levels of thyroid hormone, there are no symptoms to indicate a thyroid dysfunction. Yet, such a thyroid insufficiency raises the risk of heart disease. Thyroid replacement can lessen or eliminate this risk.

Many studies have shown when patients at risk for heart disease supplement both forms of thyroid, the T4 and T3, they experience positive results. Studies have also proven that thyroid therapy can decrease all the cardiovascular alterations influenced by hypothyroidism. By reviewing the studies and evaluating the beneficial effects of thyroid hormone, one can easily appreciate how optimal thyroid supplementation can be a very important aspect of preventive medicine.

Thyroid is a dynamic hormone with a hand in all the important processes of the body and mind. I cannot stress enough the absolute necessity to make thyroid testing (both TSH levels and free T3 and T4 levels) a part of your annual check-up regimen. Optimizing thyroid hormone levels will not only improve the way you feel and function, but also provide you with heart protection. With optimized thyroid health, your heart will only be healthier.

Thyroid and Your Hair

For years, I watched as the hair of one of my patients, Melinda, grew thinner and thinner. Every time I saw her, I asked whether she wanted to take thyroid—a minimal monthly investment for fuller hair. Each time, she turned me down because her primary care physician  told her thyroid medicine wouldn't help. So rather than have a luxurious head of hair, she lets it get thinner and thinner by the year.

The secret to combating thinning hair might be found in optimal thyroid supplementation. Most women after age 50 will experience hair thinning. As physicians, we assume it is due to androgenic hair loss. The problem is 50-year-old women don't have androgens. It is my experience that thyroid hormone might prevent hair loss and restore hair's thickness.

Why do people suffering from thyroid insufficiency lose their hair? It is believed decreased metabolism in the scalp follicles causes the head to release the hair's shaft, root and all. Hair can also become too brittle and be lost to split ends and breakage.

This is also where the difference between "normal" and "optimal" is the key. The body conserves energy whenever it can. If thyroid hormone production is not optimal, the body will shut down those functions considered non-essential—such as hair growth. If you want your hair to grow back, you'll need a higher level of thyroid hormone than normally found in your body. Even normal thyroid hormone levels may not be adequate for many women to retain hair. The hormone necessary for hair maintenance is T3. When T3 levels fall below optimal, many women will lose their hair. In particular, women on T4 preparations of Levoxyl® or Synthroid® can lose hair because these drugs don't adequately convert T4 to T3. Many doctors misdiagnose this hair loss as the result of too much thyroid when in reality it is often due to too little thyroid. Most women with thinning hair will have low T3 levels.

Hair loss might be reversed with a fairly high dose of natural thyroid medicine. One of the side effects of Synthroid® is actually prolonged or excessive hair loss. With the proper supplementation of natural thyroid hormone, optimal levels of T3 can restore healthy hair.

My Levels are Normal, but I Feel Terrible'

How many of you have actually been diagnosed with hypothyroidism? Was this a huge sigh of relief because there was finally an explanation for the fatigue, depression, absentmindedness and weight gain you have experienced? Did your doctor write you a prescription for the most popular cure, Synthroid®, and send you on your way? Do you feel better? Most likely, you do not.

> "In my view, physicians should be treating to make their patients better, not to improve their patients' TSH levels."
>
> --Alan L. Rubin, MD
> Endocrinology and Metabolism
> Private Practice

How many of you have normal blood tests (TSH/T4)? Have you read countless articles and books on hypothyroidism? Do you recognize yourself in many of the symptom descriptions? Many times I treat patients who have been labeled normal. Their TSH and T4 tests are normal. All systems, except for their symptoms, check out OK. Their doctors can't reconcile themselves to the idea of prescribing thyroid only to treat symptoms. So, their symptoms continue and are dismissed as signs of normal aging.

Mary Shoman, the thyroid guru for the layman, refers to this pandemic of overlooked symptoms as "under-treated hypothyroidism." She defines it as hypothyroidism on a cellular level. What this means is although the TSH level remains normal, the patient still suffers from such symptoms as fatigue, weight gain, depression, muscle/joint pain and hair and skin dryness. This can happen for a few reasons: the wrong medicine or the wrong diagnosis of what TSH actually indicates. The body's metabolism is directly related to the thyroid hormones' effect on the receptor site of the cells. Even if the TSH level is normal, a low T3 level or a resistant receptor site can cause the symptoms of low thyroid function. It is the lack of optimal T3 levels or ineffective stimulation of thyroid receptor sites that is primarily responsible for the signs and symptoms of hypothyroidism. Since T3 is the metabolic hormone responsible for all the thyroid action, then the emphasis should be on optimizing T3 levels as well as thyroid receptor site stimulation.

TSH levels can indicate an illness or a deficiency some of the time. I firmly believe in the importance of tests measuring free T3 and free T4. T4 levels will not always tell the truth of thyroid insufficiency, nor will TSH. The most accurate information on thyroid health is achieved with a combination of the three blood tests. TSH is an indicator of the body's need for thyroid as sensed by the hypothalamus in the brain. The hypothalamus senses low blood levels of T4 and corrects the deficiency by raising TSH levels to stimulate the thyroid gland. This will then produce more thyroid hormone. The hypothalamus does not sense low T3 levels or receptor site resistance, which is why TSH is a poor indicator of thyroid function.

Thyroid replacement carries with it tremendous health and feel-good benefits. By lecturing to medical academies all over the United States, my goal is to educate more doctors on the benefits of natural thyroid replacement. This is sometimes difficult as most of us were not taught about thyroid insufficiency in medical school. Patients frequently ask how their personal physician can become educated in prescribing natural hormones. Arming yourself with information to educate and train your doctor may not always be an effective tool. After ten years of training physicians in prescribing, monitoring, adjusting and balancing hormones, I can personally say there is much more to prescribing natural hormone replacement therapy than simply writing a prescription. Physicians usually attend an intensive two- to three- day course, which introduces them to this new trend in medicine. Convincing a physician, who is not familiar with prescribing natural hormone replacement therapy, will not be beneficial to you. If your doctor is not familiar with prescribing, monitoring, and adjusting hormones the most appropriate suggestion you can offer is for him or her to attend a training course.

What Thyroid Should I Be Taking?

This is where the heated debate arises and where I disagree with many physicians treating thyroid deficiency today. The crux of natural hormone replacement therapy is that hormones used for supplementation need to be exact replicas of what the body produces. This is essential for the body to achieve optimal results from a hormone replacement program. The most effective thyroid hormone replacements are the bio identical options, (Armour®, Westhroid® and Naturethyroid®). My preferred choice of thyroid hormone is one which is prepared or compounded by a compounding pharmacist. This natural T4 and T3 combination should be in bio identical ratios allowing for better absorption and sustained levels.

Pharmaceutical companies have financial incentives to push synthetic forms of hormone replacement. The same mindset that governs prescriptions of progesterone and estrogen also applies to thyroid.

The body naturally responds to two types of thyroid, T4 and T3. Without optimal levels from both thyroids, the body will remain deficient of thyroid hormone. The optimization of metabolism and energy production through thyroid supplementation cannot be emphasized enough. Although many doctors would agree with this desire for optimal wellness, the way they achieve maximum metabolism and energy is incorrect.

The most popular thyroids on the market today are products called Synthroid®, Levoxyl® or L-thyroxine (levothyroxine). All of these contain only T4, with the assumption T4 will convert into active T3. The pharmaceutical companies argue that these conventional synthetic forms offer a steady, more controlled hormonal level. The problem I've found with this assumption is that the T4 in Synthroid® does not readily convert into T3. Although the TSH and T4 remain at normal levels, many patients still complain of the classic symptoms of low thyroid. If doctors measured the free T3 levels on these patients', they would be surprised to find most are quite low.

Physicians have been taught to focus only on the TSH level, therefore ignoring the most important parameters which are free T3 and Free T4. It is T3 that is important at the cellular level, so it only makes sense for us to focus on optimal T3 levels instead. In addition, as physicians we have been taught that we need to only replace T4 as the body will automatically convert T4 to T3. We are taught that if the body needs T3, it will make enough. Unfortunately, this is not the case. The body makes less and less T3 as we get older. Almost all women over 50 will have free T3 levels in the lower 15 percent of normal. This is due to the fact the body converts less and less T4 into T3.

The history of natural thyroid is a long one. It has been used for decades, as early as 1892. For the longest time, it was the only form of therapy for hypothyroidism. Since T3 has a short half-life, doctors shied away from its use and instead chose the "safer and more controllable" T4.

Synthroid® quickly became the "in" thyroid. It was backed by a large and profitable pharmaceutical company; studies were conducted in its favor so why not prescribe this drug. In the meantime, natural thyroid lost its significance and doctors referred to it as outdated.

Since Synthroid® hit the mainstream market, I've noticed many patients fighting with a thyroid deficiency. They take Synthroid® religiously every morning, but often with minimal effect. The FDA actually fined Knoll Pharmaceutics $90 million for forging research findings and withholding truthful, but disastrous results, from other studies. The purpose was to convince physicians and patients that Synthroid® was better than the "outdated" natural thyroid.

I assessed the above claims in my own study of patients with normal TSH levels, some on Synthroid® and some not. All patients had the classic symptoms of hypothyroidism: decreased energy, slower thought processes, and hair and skin changes. In our two clinical studies, we came to the conclusion that T4 alone, as seen in products like Synthroid® and Levoxyl®, does not adequately convert into T3 and consequently cannot result in symptomatic improvement.

It is important to understand that as we age, thyroid insufficiency results from:

- Decreased production of T4
- Decreased conversion of T4 into T3
- Decreased sensitivity of receptor sites

Thereby, any one of these three age-related thyroid complications can cause symptoms.

Some of these patients are not necessarily clinically ill or symptomatic. Their thyroid function is simply not optimal.

184

Synthetic T4 medications (Synthroid®, Levoxyl®, and Thyroxine) rarely, if ever, adequately convert into T3. T3 is the true protagonist of the body's health and metabolism. As a doctor, I took an oath to do no harm. My patients' optimal well-being is my first priority; pleasing the public is my last.

How to be Heard

Simply listen to the patient. They will eventually tell you what the diagnosis is.
—A wise professor from medical school.

Because hypothyroidism can cause undesired weight gain, skin texture changes, body temperature dips, fatigue, depression, and cardiac complications, it is especially important for you and your doctor to become acquainted with your thyroid hormone levels. They must be optimized for maximum health benefit.

Preventive medicine is more cost effective and it saves lives. Think about it: you could stop heart disease before it starts, you could maintain your active lifestyle well into your twilight years and you could keep your mind and emotions in check. These elemental facets of good health largely depend on the thyroid gland. They are regulated throughout your life by sufficient thyroid levels. As you get older, they decline. If you maintain them at optimal levels, you will not suffer the consequences of thyroid insufficiency.

Maintaining your health makes a rather good case for a yearly check-up. It is up to you to take a preventive approach to your long-term well being. I personally chose the preventive approach and have never looked back.

In Short...

Thyroid's Benefits: Thyroid hormone results in increased metabolism, temperature and warmth. It increases fat breakdown, resulting in weight loss as well as lower cholesterol. It protects against cardiovascular disease, improves cerebral metabolism, and prevents cognitive impairment. Low thyroid hormone causes thin sparse hair, dry skin, and thin nails. Low thyroid levels also cause fatigue and depression.

Thyroid's Side Effects: Large doses in sensitive patients can cause sweating, tremors, and palpitations. Utilizing correct doses and monitoring patients can prevent these mild side effects.

The Bottom Line: You don't have to slow down. You can replace your thyroid hormone to the optimal levels they once were in your 20s or 30s (not just normal levels, as the more orthodox medical field would advise). As with other hormones, there are many health and feel good benefits.

Melatonin: The Aging Loophole

After my hysterectomy I started waking up on
and off at night and found that several nights
a week I never fell completely asleep. I couldn't
function during the day and felt on edge. My
friend had a bottle of melatonin and gave me a
week's supply. The first night I took it, I slept
fantastic, and what's more incredible is that I
never had to take prescription sleep aids—I
could find relief in something natural to my
body's chemistry.
—Jamie, 54

Aging doesn't have to be as rough as it's made out to be. Scientists and doctors have isolated a molecule that has many important health benefits and also makes us feel and function at our best. What is this molecule? It's a hormone that is a naturally-occurring sleep aid, a hormone that is an essential part of the longevity equation.

Read more!

The best-known, most comprehensive book on this hormone is *The Melatonin Miracle* by the researchers and doctors, William Regelson and Walter Pierpaoli. It's 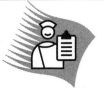 a must-read for anyone curious about the ongoing discoveries being made regarding melatonin's functional importance in the human body.

Melatonin, a natural sleep aid which people have taken for years, is the hormone that first opened physicians' eyes to the possibility of successfully preventing age-related illness.

Researchers have been investigating it since 1958 and have recently uncovered remarkable benefits.

Scientists have been able to demonstrate that melatonin can slow the aging process in animals with genetic make-ups similar to that of humans—indicating it can have the same benefits for us. Because of the powerful evidence reaped from these studies, researchers are now looking into melatonin's potential as a powerful antioxidant, cancer inhibitor, immune system booster, and the positive effects it may have on ailments such as heart disease, AIDS, Alzheimer's disease, and Parkinson's disease. Up-to-date research shows the potential of this hormone may be vast in both its immediate and long-term benefits.

Melatonin isn't just a sleep enhancer anymore! This chapter is going to explore five of the far-reaching effects:

- Sleep aid
- Mood enhancer
- Immune system booster
- Cancer inhibitor
- Treatment for blood pressure and migraine headaches

Let's Get Technical: Melatonin

Melatonin is derived from a chain of events starting with an amino acid called tryptophan. Tryptophan is synthesized into serotonin, which by the action of two enzymes is catalyzed into melatonin.

Once melatonin is released by the pineal gland, it goes into the local blood stream and then into the body's blood circulation where it has access to every bodily fluid and tissue. Its production is influenced primarily by the night-and-day cycle: in the light, production of melatonin decreases; with darkness, melatonin levels rise dramatically, causing us to become drowsy.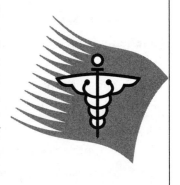

Interestingly, unlike most hormones, melatonin does not necessarily need a receptor site; melatonin's small molecular structure and solubility allow it to permeate almost every cell in the body. Therefore, more than just a natural tranquilizer, melatonin seems to affect all organs and systems.

Melatonin can help you create a new medical paradigm for healthy, vibrant aging. As you probe deeper into how to preserve your own well-being, you'll soon learn hormone replacement in general (and melatonin in particular) is looked upon in many important ways. As you read about the many researchers and their numerous studies backing up the potential application of melatonin, you will find the many health and feel-good benefits. Evidence published in some of the most prestigious medical journals demonstrates improved quality of living and healthier aging through supplementation of melatonin.

Perhaps most importantly, melatonin has proven itself—since 1958—to be necessary and *safe*. Studies have proved its efficacy. The benefits far outweigh any possible side effects. Side effects may include sleepiness when a dose is too high. This can be eliminated by lowering the dose.

Some doctors are cautious about hormone replacement of any kind because of the association with "alternative medicine." Many reputable scientific studies support hormone replacement therapy and its relationship to healthy aging. In the case of melatonin, there are more than 50 years of studies bolstering its safety in several clinical applications. If 50 years isn't considered long term, what is? The lack of melatonin in the body clearly may cause harm.

As melatonin production decreases with age, so do our regular sleep patterns. Any disruption in our quality of sleep and deep stages of sleep will adversely affect our immune system and overall health. Maintaining adequate melatonin levels helps to avoid many age-related ailments. More importantly and most recently, medical research has demonstrated melatonin's important role in both cancer prevention and treatment.

Nature's Little Pacemaker

Let's return for a moment to the technical definition of melatonin. It is produced in the pineal gland—a tiny, pine-cone-shaped gland tucked deep within the human brain. Once thought of as an evolutionary leftover, it was discovered that the pineal gland controls many bodily functions.

As melatonin production drops, our sleep cycle becomes irregular, which influences immune health and

190

hormonal secretion. Melatonin is a crucial ingredient in the recipe for feeling young. It is important to maintain an ongoing supply of this hormone produced by a youthful pineal gland. This important hormone is optimized by supplementing the body with melatonin. Many documented studies, from laboratories around the world, have confirmed the powerful link between the functions/secretions of the pineal gland and longevity.

Like other hormones, melatonin can't stop time, but it can derail or delay many of time's debilitating effects. It may not be the most glamorous hormone, but it is a necessary addition for anyone who is serious about health maintenance. Melatonin is the hormone leading us toward healthier aging by boosting immune function.

Sleep: Nature's Tonic

Sometimes the best medicine is simply a good night's rest. Sleep has its own regenerating power that can do wonders at reconstructing the damage done during the waking hours. The only rest for the senses is deep sleep, and the only way to fall into that stage IV sleep is through the ebb and flow of melatonin. The lackluster sleep we experience as we get older influences our health in noticeable ways — bad concentration and irritable moods.

The pineal gland is wired to a paired cluster of nerve cells above the optic chasm in the hypothalamus. At night, darkness sends a message to this cluster of nerves, which then sends impulses to the pineal gland, which in turn, secretes melatonin.

Melatonin causes the yawning, the droopy eyelids, the heavy limbs, and the yearning to curl up under the covers and sleep. Its levels rise tenfold at night, peaking at around two in the morning and enhancing stage IV sleep. This is the deepest sleep, where the body and mind recoup from daily stresses.

Out of motivation to get a good night's sleep, I personally take melatonin. All of its other benefits are just bonuses. I have noticed that as I get older, sleep is not as easy to come by. I find myself tossing and turning without the aid of melatonin. Throughout the next day, I have a more difficult time focusing and concentrating.

> Sleep is essential to staying healthy and happy and melatonin is the elixir to a good night's rest.

Melatonin induces a deep sleep, which allows our bodies and minds to stay healthy. Laymen's proof of this is seen in our reaction to tossing and turning at night. Nights of sleeplessness can drastically inhibit our immune system and can also inhibit our sense of humor and goodwill to others. Sleep is essential to staying healthy and happy. Melatonin is the elixir to a good night's rest.

With age comes a drop in melatonin production. With this drop comes insomnia and sleep disorders. Lack of sleep can add to the stresses on the body and the immune system. This contributes problems associated with aging. Supplementing with melatonin can be an effective treatment for insomnia in older patients.

Because melatonin controls circadian rhythms, it can also reset the sleep cycle when it gets interrupted. Travelers have used melatonin for years to fight jet lag. By taking melatonin the first night you arrive in a new time zone, the circadian rhythm is forced to adjust at a faster rate. The few days of vacation you've always set aside for "zombie-mode" can now be open to a world of opportunities.

Throughout the United States, many people depend upon prescription sleep aids to get through the night. These types of sleep aids can have side effects, and can become addictive. Melatonin is a safe, powerful and non-addictive hormone.

Recently, the FDA approved a new drug to treat insomnia, Rozerem®. It stimulates the melatonin receptors. Why purchase an expensive drug when you can take an inexpensive, natural supplement? Rather than take a drug that stimulates the melatonin receptors, why not simply supplement with melatonin? It is a safer, inexpensive, tremendously beneficial hormone designed to be there in the first place.

Keeping our Immune System Strong

The key to preventing illness is to keep our immune system operating in top form. The strength of our immune system directly affects how our body fends off foreign invaders, from a simple flu bug to cancer cells. As we age, if we do not practice preventive medicine our immune system begins its own decline. As this process occurs, it becomes much more difficult to ward off common ailments like the flu or colds.

How is the absence of melatonin related to the decline in our immune system? Studies on animals have repeatedly shown that when the pineal gland is removed and melatonin synthesis is inhibited, the subjects experienced a form of immunosuppression. Yet, when melatonin is restored orally, a healthy immune system is jump-started.

Melatonin supplementation helps shore up our defenses on both fronts by improving our immune system's memory and strengthening antibody response. This allows our immune system to function closer to the peak level we once had.

Many studies support that melatonin may be successfully used in the therapy of immunosupressed conditions. There is also evidence melatonin can help restore thymus function and enhance T-cell production. By enhancing T-cell production, melatonin helps the body fight viruses – another vital factor in maintaining optimal function of the immune system.

> Melatonin can help alleviate the effects and damage from stressors in our environment and be an important, natural tranquilizer.

T-cells and the thymus gland work to help eliminate the negative side effects of stress. When you're stressed, your susceptibility to infection heightens. The immune system breaks down under the pressure of chronic stress and the body opens up to a world of common colds and flues.

Melatonin can regulate the production of T-cells. Melatonin also augments the substances in the human body that lessen pain and allow our bodies to cope and heal.

Stress is nothing to take lightly. While each passing decade adds new stresses to the old, many of our natural defenses deteriorate. Melatonin, which initially protected our immune system and enhanced the benefits of our endorphins (anti-pain and anti-anxiety chemicals), suddenly decreases with added stress. Melatonin can help alleviate the damage from stressors in our environment.

Beyond melatonin's power as an immune-system booster, it is also being touted as a powerful antioxidant. A 2001 study showed melatonin's awesome free radical scavenging capabilities may help the mind as well as the body. Antioxidants are vital in combating what are known as free radicals. Free radicals are unstable molecules that attack stable molecules in order to provide themselves with the electron they are missing. Although the life span of a free radical is short, its damage can be long lasting. Some doctors and scientists believe free radicals are the direct cause of aging as they rip electrons from perfectly functioning atoms, causing degradation and disruption within a cell.

Let's Get Technical: Antioxidants and Melatonin

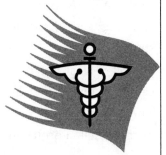

Antioxidants like vitamin E, vitamin C, glutathione, and melatonin block free radicals from robbing electrons from healthy atoms. Melatonin scavenges oxygen-centered free radicals and among the more powerful antioxidants, melatonin has been found to be the best hydroxyl scavenger. The hydroxyl radical is highly toxic and melatonin works by attaching to it to neutralize it by a single electron transfer resulting in a detoxified radical.

It's important to note here that melatonin's actions as a free radical scavenger are not mediated by receptors, and this is why I call it the hormone-of-all-trades—it has actions above and beyond the duty of a hormone.

DNA is the map of our design and suffers the most from ionizing radiation due to oxidative stress. Melatonin shields the macromolecules such as DNA from injury, halting the proliferation of degenerative changes.

Because melatonin flows so easily in and out of cellular compartments, it is a constant and potent antioxidant. Melatonin, in fact, may guard against a number of conditions tied to oxidative stress like Alzheimer's Disease, Cancer, Parkinson's Disease, Multiple Sclerosis and Rheumatoid Arthritis.

Melatonin has many receptor sites in the human brain. Studies have revealed that it may have a definitive purpose as a natural defense in many age-related degenerative diseases. Of course, its antioxidant applications are clear. Whether we can use this knowledge to fight off diseases like Parkinson's and Alzheimer's has yet to be seen. Fighting free-radical damage is the beginning in our quest for a healthier aging. Melatonin's worth in this arena is indisputable.

Where we stand with melatonin and other hormones regarding age-related diseases is still under investigation. The supplementation of some hormones has been proven to protect against age related degeneration. As for melatonin, I can only report the direction in which studies are pointing. The conclusions from these studies suggest melatonin is instrumental in protecting our health in many different ways.

Cancer—A Common Foe of Aging

Because melatonin augments the immune response and battles against free radicals, it is no surprise it is also believed to be an inhibitor of tumor growth. It acts as a mediator to many other hormones and helps protect against cancers. Melatonin has been shown to indirectly attack breast cancer cells and impede prostate cancer cells. It is useful as a supplement in cancer therapy.

Melatonin's cancer-obstructing benefits, along with its therapeutic benefits, are being studied by cancer research centers. We can only conclude from the large amount of data that melatonin has a place in this field of research. A plethora of studies have proven melatonin's multiple effects in treating cancer and lessening the side effects of chemotherapy. Most currently, melatonin is being touted as an important adjunct in protecting against breast cancer. The studies listed in this book pose a good case when it comes to using melatonin to treat cancer and other diseases.

Is Melatonin for You?

Melatonin has proven to be one of the safest hormones you can take. Tests administering high doses to both mice and humans have indicated no toxic effects. In January 1997, the *New England Journal of Medicine* published the most extensive review of melatonin yet to appear in a conventional medical journal. This article extolled melatonin's powerful antioxidant effects, including its potential for treating and preventing cancer, its immuno-enhancing properties, its potential as an antioxidant, and its power to induce better sleep and treat jet lag.

Melatonin is supported by multiple peer-reviewed studies. These studies are featured in some of the world's most prestigious medical journals and have demonstrated the efficacy of melatonin.

In Short…

Melatonin's Benefits: Melatonin helps boost the immune system, fights cancers, alleviates some symptoms of harsh cancer treatments, and acts as a natural sleep aid.

Melatonin's Side Effects: Melatonin is extremely safe and non-toxic. A few users have experienced headaches or grogginess with higher doses. The dose of melatonin is adjusted based on sleep parameters.

The Bottom Line: Melatonin is a vital component to both the endocrine and immune systems. It is key to the maintenance of the thymus gland and T-cell production, antibody effectiveness, circadian rhythm, and a powerful free radical scavenger. Most importantly, melatonin is one of the hormones shown time and again to prevent age-associated deterioration and may protect against age-related disease.

Epilogue:
Making the Choice for a Healthy Longevity

Two of my patients, a husband and wife, sent me a postcard from the Caribbean where they were vacationing for a month. They wrote: "Enjoying the sun, enjoying each other, enjoying our seventies...Thanks." A simple statement, but packed with so much meaning. As you read this book, the most important understanding you will have is through natural hormone replacement therapy, you can truly begin to enjoy the remaining years in your life. Whether you are forty-five or sixty-four or eighty-nine, it's never too late to discover healthy aging. Remember—it's not the years in your life, it's the life in your years!

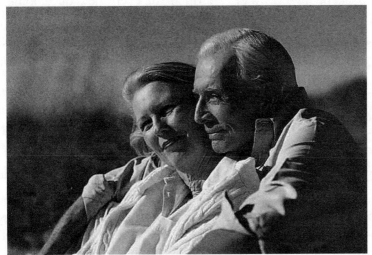

USA Today Snapshots features contemporary trivia about how we, as a nation, feel about our healthcare and culture. In a "snapshot" *USA Today* tallied the biggest concerns Americans have about growing older. The number one fear, 83%, was the "slowing down" effects associated with aging. Following closely at 81% was an unease regarding "overall health," and at 56%, many people worried about becoming a "family burden." This book started out with my personal journey into healthier aging. Like many others, I recognized my own downward spiral was imminent. I felt the first stings of aging at forty-three and agonized over slowing down, losing my health and burdening my family. These concerns spurred me to become my own personal guinea pig in an experiment I hoped would reap a more fruitful future. Lucky for me, I succeeded. I realized my own experiences were not reason enough for me to feel secure in prescribing hormones to my patients. In truth, I wanted to share with the whole world just how great I felt. Instead, I delved into medical texts and journals, stockpiled studies past and present, and kept my eyes and ears open for every new development on the horizon. The proof was monumental - our quality of life, our health, and our happiness seemingly dwindle at the same rate our hormone levels decline. As we restore each hormone to optimal levels, our body and mind will again enjoy the health, vigor and vitality we once possessed. This conclusion is apparent in the many studies outlined in the chapters of this book. Our hormones keep us healthy and when restored to optimal levels, they keep us youthful and energetic. This was reason enough to devote my life and medical knowledge to the health and well-being of every patient.

Where We Stand Today

We live on the cusp of a new science and medicine. This new field is something I began working in long before it became as popular as it is today. The baby boomers and their offspring are a lucky group of people. They live in a world of ever changing perceptions about aging. Undeniably, we will often be confronted with negative outlooks that present aging as something unavoidable. However, with a little help from the media, I am sure you will continue to familiarize yourself with the new attitude. Television and magazines like Time or Newsweek will keep you on the cusp with new and exciting articles. Aging and its related complexities are being transformed from a normal way of life into something positive through healthy living and supplementation of natural 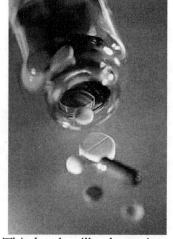 hormones, vitamins, and minerals. This book will substantiate many of the popular claims the media brings to the forefront. It is packed with hardcore evidence from prestigious medical journals and from my own experiences as a doctor. The doors are now opened to the possibility of healthy aging for years to come. Seize this opportunity to optimize your fifties, sixties, seventies and beyond with the same passion and energy you enjoyed throughout your twenties and thirties.

Although there is ample clinical data compiled in this book regarding the benefits of natural hormone replacement, there is a prevalence of fear in our mainstream culture. It is instigated more out of ignorance than genuine insight. Therefore, I would like to venture a rebuttal to the negative news about the whole spectrum of longevity medicine. As a well-educated and curious reader, my first warning is that articles concerning hormone replacement are usually centered on chemically-altered hormones, like Provera® or Premarin®. It cannot be implied that molecularly altered hormones will have the same outcome as natural hormones which are created to fit human receptor sites like a lock and key mechanism.

Hormones have kept you healthy thus far and deductive reasoning supports the conclusion that supplementing with the exact replica would result in the 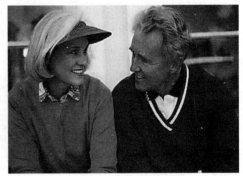 same healthy effect. As hormones take a plunge at menopause, a woman's susceptibility to heart disease and osteoporosis increase tremendously. Studies demonstrate how men over fifty gain visceral fat and lose muscle, both leading them down the road to heart disease. Experts have overlooked the landmark studies, which prove through meta-analysis or double blind placebo-controlled trials that testosterone, estrogen, progesterone and thyroid naturally create an environment for living longer and living better.

Through this book, I give you the hope that doctors and patients will recognize there is a choice in how we age.

Science has revealed women and men can remain healthy, happy and dynamic late in life with optimal hormone supplementation. The resigned attitude toward aging is now turning to one of hope and anticipation. Use this book as a catalyst, a starting point and a tool. Let it inspire you to share with your doctor the need for an all-inclusive approach to preventive medicine. Instead of waiting for an age-related illness to occur, take a proactive approach and practice prevention. We live in a time when great scientific leaps are being made. Let's get a handle on how we age. We have a choice and the choice is natural hormone replacement therapy.

Pharmacies of the Past, Reshaping the Future

Compounding Pharmacies are a select group of United States' pharmacies providing customized pharmaceutical products. Conscientious practitioners and patients no longer need to settle for mass-produced medication in limited dosages and routes of administration. To provide for your specific needs, compounding pharmacies blend time-honored techniques of individual formulation with modern medical knowledge and stringent quality control. Pharmacies you find in your local neighborhood serve generalities, not particulars. They

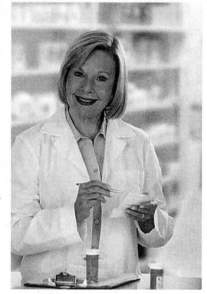

serve a purpose of convenience and most of your normal pharmaceutical needs—antibiotics, anti-depressants, pain medication, or common cold cures. But natural hormone replacement therapy depends on an entirely precise mixture which big pharmaceutical companies cannot afford to worry about. Titration of hormone levels and matching medications to create an optimal therapy for each individual person is the specialty of a compounding pharmacy. Pharmaceutical companies cannot patent natural hormones without molecularly altering their structure. These alterations cause side effects to come into the picture. Because you are unique, what your body needs and how your body will react to certain doses of a particular hormone is also unique. Therefore, it is important to find a compounding pharmacy with the capability of making hormones to match individual variance and to do so with bio-identical hormones.

So, first things first--find a doctor and program that suit your personal health care needs. Find a pharmacy you can trust. There are several compounding pharmacies in America which specialize in creating bio-identical hormones. They can formulate the exact dosage your doctor prescribes for you. If you're having difficulty finding a doctor comfortable with prescribing natural hormones, I have a few suggestions. If you find a compounding pharmacy near you, contact the pharmacist and ask for a referral to a practitioner who has prescribed natural hormones through them. If unsuccessful, contact one of the larger compounding pharmacies that ship nationally. **MedQuest Pharmacy** serves practitioners across the country and also has a list of physicians who have been through my hormone training course; this is a good place to start. They can be reached online at www.mqrx.com or by phone at 888.222.2956. For information about becoming a patient of mine, visit www.hormonedoc.com.

Are You Ready?

So, the question is, are you ready to regain your youth? Are you ready to assume your future with the knowledge and wisdom your age suggests, without the wrinkles, the weakness and the ailments? A hormone replacement program that is natural and tailored to your exacting needs can offer you that kind of aging— one manifested by 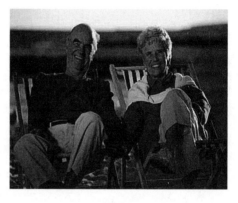 glowing health and dynamism. With the supplementation of thyroid, testosterone, melatonin, and DHEA (and the addition of estrogen and progesterone if you are female), you can enjoy the promise of healthy aging. The cliché "happiness truly comes from within" is not too far from the truth. With hormones in their optimal range, our beauty and energy can resurface, and possibilities can reawaken. I encourage you to push the aging envelope. Discover that magical, elusive fountain of youth with ingredients your body has understood since its very conception—hormones.

Let this book awaken your curiosity. Let this book be the foundation of your rebirth into the next half of your life. The time is now to shake the stereotype of old age and regain the confidence you've worked hard to possess. Natural hormone replacement therapy holds the key to unraveling the mystery to a longer, healthier, and more enjoyable future.

The Scientific Justification for Bio Identical Hormones: A Literature Review and Bibliography with Comments From Neal Rouzier, M.D.

This is my favorite chapter from the standpoint that it provides scientific justification for all that I preach concerning optimal replacement of bio identical hormones. The most important quotes from our most prestigious medical journals are listed, followed by my personal thoughts and commentary. After reading this chapter, there should not be one physician that should not understand and embrace this therapy, both for themselves and their patients. NR

By the nature of the beast, doctors always demand proof and efficacy of any treatment or therapy. We as physicians are extremely critical of any new therapy and will critique any medicine or procedure until we are convinced of the safety and efficacy through well-designed medical studies. However, while a therapy may be well substantiated in the medical literature, the old dictum of "if a doctor is not up on something, then he is down on it," certainly holds true.

For those of you who wish to provide evidence from the medical literature to your friends and physicians, then these reference articles are for you. A physician once asked me if I could prove that these natural hormones were as good as the synthetic hormones. I asked him in return if he could prove the synthetic hormones were as good as the natural hormones. I can provide hundreds of articles demonstrating the harmful effects of the synthetic hormones, and I can provide hundreds of articles revealing the deterioration that our bodies experience with loss of our own hormones. The following are direct quotes from our medical literature that acknowledge the benefits of hormones, the harm and deterioration that occur when hormone levels fall, and the harmful effects that occur when utilizing non bio identical, chemically altered hormones.

As I stated previously, our own hormones are not harmful to our body. The harm is when our hormone levels fall – that is when we deteriorate and suffer loss of strength, energy, libido, structure, muscle and bone. That's when we see a decrease in quality of life and an increase in lassitude and depression. Worst of all is the increase in heart disease, strokes, osteoporosis, Alzheimer's and dementia. I find it amazing that over 40 years of medical studies that support the benefits of hormones remain ignored. The following are quotes from our prestigious medical journals that should not be ignored.

General Hormone Replacement Therapy

"Aging is not an unalterable process of decline and loss. Hormones are now responsible for this change in attitude. Therefore, routine medical intervention programs offering long-term replacement therapy with one or more hormones to delay the aging process, allowing us to live for a longer period in a relatively intact state, are becoming popular."

Biomedicina 2000 Jan;Vol 3(1):6-7.

(This is appropriately termed preventive medicine or age management medicine.)

(Although many people have an appropriate fear of HRT, this comes from media hype and the medical studies demonstrating the harm of the synthetic hormones. Do not extrapolate this to include natural hormones.)

"Hormone replacement prevents weight gain. HRT favors weight loss by increasing lipid oxidation, improving insulin response and lowering plasma lipids." *Maturitas 1999 Aug;16 32(3): 147 -53*.
(All studies show beneficial effects, except those studies evaluating synthetic hormones.)

DHEA

"DHEA increases insulin sensitivity, decreases abdominal fat, prevents and treats the metabolic syndrome and thereby prevents diabetes." *JAMA 2004;292: 2243-2248*.
(All hormones have beneficial health effects and replacing them to optimal levels guarantees this benefit.)

"High DHEA levels are related to lower carotid intimal wall thickness." *J Clin Endocrinol Metab 1999 June;84(6):2008-12*

"DHEA was found to be beneficial in treating Lupus patients. DHEA was well tolerated without side effects." *J Rheumatology 1998;25(2):285-9*.

"DHEA treats depression and improves memory. DHEA lowered cortisol levels." *Biological Psychiatry 1997;41(3):311-8*.

"DHEA decreases heart disease and atherosclerosis." *Annals N.Y. Academy of Science: 1995 Dec;774:271-280.*

"High levels of DHEA decrease mortality from heart disease. Low levels of DHEA are associated with increased mortality. The higher the DHEA, the better the protection against mortality from any cause." *New England Journal of Medicine 1986 Dec;315(24):1519-24.*

"DHEA blocks carcinogenesis. Low levels of DHEA demonstrate an increased risk of cancer and cardiovascular disease." *Journal of Clinical Invest 1988 August;82(2);712-720.*

"DHEA caused a remarkable increase in physical and psychological well-being. There were no side effects and DHEA was well tolerated." *Journal of Clinical Endrocrinology Metab 1997 June;78(6):1360-7.*

"DHEA restores well-being, increases bone density and decreases vaginal dryness." *Journal Clinical Endocrinology Metab. 1997 Oct;82(10):3498-505.*

"DHEA treatment for significant anti-depressant effects." *American Journal of Psychiatry 1999;150:646-649.*
(All HRT has health benefits and DHEA is no different. There are many benefits for cardiovascular, psychiatric, musculoskeletal and genitourinary systems. Improvement in well-being and depression has been well demonstrated.)

"DHEA administration reduces abdominal fat, decreases insulin resistance and protects against metabolic syndrome and diabetes." *JAMA 2004 November; Vol.292(18):2233-2247.*

"Low DHEA levels are associated with depression and depressed mood." *J American Gerentology Soc.1999 June;47(6):685-91.*

"DHEA is beneficial in treatment of major depression in women." *Am. J Psychiatry 1999 April;156(4):646-649.*

"DHEA improves mood and fatigue." *J Psych 2000 Dec;85(12):4650-56.*

"DHEA improves well-being, sexuality, and cognition." *Endocrinology Research. 2000 Nov;26(4):505*

"DHEA improves immune function and decreases mortality." *Critical Care Med. 2001Feb;29(2):380*

"DHEA improves strength and body composition." *Clinical Endocrinology 1998 Oct;49 (4)421-32.*

"DHEA reduces LDL cholesterol and body fat." *Journal Family Med 1988 Jan;60(1): 57-61.*

"Epidemiologic studies demonstrate that low levels of DHEA increase risk of cancer, heart disease, immune dysfunction, diabetes, and obesity. "DHEA replacement increases bone density, improves depression, cognition, sexual function." *Am J Health Syst. Pharm; 57(22):2048-2056*

"The goal of replacement therapy is to restore DHEA to the upper level of normal of a young adult range. Those patients experience a reduction in fatigue, improvement in mood and psychological well-being." *J Clin Endomet. 1994 June;78(6):1360-67*

211

Estrogen

"There is an impressive, large collection of biological data and observational studies indicating that postmenopausal HRT protects against heart disease and stroke. There is good reason to believe that the full impact of estrogen's beneficial actions on cardiovascular tissue requires the presence of healthy endothelium (normal blood vessels). It is most appropriate to prescribe hormones to post menopausal women to protect against cardiovascular disease. Vascular biologists are convinced of estrogen's essential role in protecting against cardiovascular disease. Estrogen's role is protecting against the development of atherosclerosis." *Circulation 2001;104:499-503.*

> (Estrogen should be taken by all women starting at menopause and continued indefinitely. The term estrogen denotes bio identical estrogen.)

"This manuscript presents a protocol for hormone replacement therapy with natural estradiol, progesterone, testosterone, DHEA and melatonin. Using the natural sex steroids which occur naturally in humans represents replacement to ensure attainment of pre-menopausal levels and adequacy of therapy. This is inexpensive therapy that gives relief of symptoms, is well tolerated, provides minimal side effects, protects the endometrium, and results in excellent compliance. This replacement of natural hormones is based on sound physiologic principles that have been demonstrated to be the preferred method of hormone replacement." *Infertility and Reproductive Medicine Clinics of North America; 1995 October; Vol. 6 (4):653-675.*

> (This article was one of the first of many articles to appear in our medical literature that researched the efficacy and superiority of bio identical hormones. It is a classic article demonstrating the importance of natural

hormones and the harm and side effects of synthetic hormones. Although many people have an appropriate fear of HRT, this comes from media hype and the medical studies demonstrating the harm of the synthetic hormones. Do not extrapolate this to include natural hormones. This study provides credence that it is the synthetic hormones that cause the harmful effects and not the natural hormones.)

"Fear of breast cancer is the strongest factor limiting postmenopausal hormone use. The most powerful study to date definitively demonstrated that estrogen does not cause an increased risk for cancer. The increased risk was associated only with taking the progestin (Provera®) and not estrogen." *JAMA 2004;291(24): 2947-2958.*

"Hormone users had an overall 50% decrease in illness and death. Estrogen reduces mood swings, depression, hot flashes, heart disease, strokes, Alzheimer's, osteoporosis, urogenital atrophy, tooth loss, macular degeneration and memory loss. Estrogen decreases overall morbidity, mortality and improves quality of life." *Hospital Practice 1999 August;295-305.*

(If women were to read the medical literature and come to realize what truly happens to their body's and health when they lose estrogen, I can't imagine that any woman would be without it.)

"Loss of hormones at menopause results in significant genital atrophy, vaginal dryness, introital stenosis, and painful intercourse." *Family Practice News 2005 March;58-59*

(I can't imagine any man not wanting his wife to be on estrogen if he truly realizes the consequences.)

"Estrogen deficiency greatly increases mortality from cardiovascular disease and osteoporosis. Over 90% of women will die from cardiovascular disease which estrogen can prevent." Over 40 years of study have well documented the cardiovascular protective effects of estrogen." *Obstet Gynecol 1996 Jan;87(1):6-12*

(How can doctors, patients, and our government ignore this?)

"The potential lethal consequences of osteoporosis are overwhelming. Estrogen is protective but only when certain serum levels are maintained." *Female Patient Oct. 2004;Vol. 29:40-46.*

(Most doctors never measure or don't know how to interpret hormone levels. Your hormone levels must be monitored and maintained to assure benefit. That which you are taking might otherwise be worthless. Over 90% of the women that come to see me that are taking "natural hormones" have estradiol levels in the dangerously low range. They might as well have been taking nothing.)

"Multiple medical studies have demonstrated estrogen's protective effects against Alzheimer's, memory loss, loss of cognition.
-Estrogen decreases colorectal cancer.
-Estrogen decreases cataracts and macular degeneration.
-Estrogen prevents tooth loss and gingivitis.
-Estrogen prevents urogenital atrophy, painful intercourse and stress incontinence."
Biomedica Jan. 2000; Vol. 3(1):6-9

(Again, patients should be told the harm of estrogen deficiency.)

"All women on natural estrogen and progesterone had a decrease in cholesterol and increase in HDL. Women on synthetic HRT had no improvement in cholesterol and many side effects. Natural HRT resulted in symptomatic improvement, an improved lipid profile, and no side effects." *Obstetrics Gynecology 1989 April; 73:606-611*

> (This was one of the very first articles to prove natural hormones are better than synthetic hormones.)

"Long term estrogen use is associated with lower mortality rate primarily through reduction in cardiovascular disease." *Obstetrics Gynecology 1996 Jan;87(1):6-12.*

> (Therefore all women that want to live longer should have optimal estrogen levels. Notice that I did not say that they should be on estrogen because taking estrogen does not guarantee protective levels. The physician must document and assure adequate blood levels; otherwise hormone replacement is worthless.)

"We must not forget the dangers of menopause and the deleterious consequences of estrogen deficiency. Estrogen protects bone, heart, brain, blood vessels, urogenital tissue, teeth, eyes. Observational data from around the world show estrogen has beneficial effects on mortality from all causes." *Consultant 2001July;Vol. 71:1085-1086*

"Estrogen, along with natural progesterone, reduces plaque formation and heart disease." *Circulation 1998 Sept;98(12):1158-63.*

> (The hormones are synergistic with one another.)

"Recent studies have identified a protective affect of estrogen in the development of Alzheimer's disease and new studies show that testosterone may exert an even stronger preventive effect." *National Academy of Science USA 1997;94:6612-6617.*

> (Multiple studies demonstrated that Alzheimer's disease can be prevented and the grave economic impact lessened. Many patients are told to stop their HRT, which increases their risk of Alzheimer's. If estrogen is started early at menopause there is an 80% decrease in Alzheimer's disease. The WHI study showed an increase in AD but only when estrogen was started after age 65. Stopping estrogen could result in millions more cases of AD.)

"Estrogen lowers cortisol which in turn reduces abdominal fat." *Female Patient April 2001;26:18-24.*

> (Estrogen, testosterone, DHEA – all lower cortisol levels, thereby reducing abdominal fat, thereby reducing diabetes and heart disease.)

> (HRT provides positive effects for women such as improved mood, improved sense of well-being, relief of urogenital atrophy, and improved bone density. Optimal benefit is obtained when estrogen is begun early in menopause and continued indefinitely.

> HRT improves bone mineral density and decreases fracture regardless of the age at which it is initiated. It is never too late to initiate HRT.)

"Bone density is rapidly lost when HRT is stopped. HRT should be continued indefinitely." *JAMA 2002 August;Vol. 288 No. 7:880-887.*

> (I could not have said it any better.)

"The largest study to date, the Nurses' Health Study, demonstrated a 100% decrease in heart disease and cancer for estrogen users. It is never too late to initiate estrogen therapy to arrest the progression of osteoporosis and hip fractures." *Female Patient 2004 Oct;Vol 29: 35-41.*

> (Pooled data from 30 trials demonstrated that HRT is associated with a reduction in total mortality of 40%. The Nurses' Health Study demonstrated significant reductions in cardiac events and total mortality. HRT can halt the progression of atherosclerosis if HRT is started early in the course of disease and near to menopause.)

"In the final analysis of the estrogen only arm of the WHI, there was no increased risk of breast cancer or heart disease. There was a 35% decrease in hip fractures, 35% decrease in diabetes and a 60% decrease in urinary sepsis. This leads to a significant decrease in all causes of mortality. *J Gen Internal Medicine 2004;19(7): 791-804*

> (Women are always afraid of breast cancer and estrogen alone has been shown not to increase the risk of breast cancer. Not taking estrogen significantly increases overall mortality from multiple other causes and most women and doctors remain oblivious to this.)

"New findings in four recent studies counter the results of WHI and HERS. Estrogen replacement results in a dramatic decrease in cardiovascular disease. Coronary artery disease deaths were not reported in the 6,000 women taking estrogen. The results of the WHI do not apply to younger women." *Family Practice News 2003 June;Vol 33(11):1-2.*

> (So many women stopped HRT as a result of the WHI study and recent studies prove the WHI results to be incorrect.)

"Estrogen reduces the incidence of Alzheimer's disease by 50%." *JAMA 2002; 288:2123-2129.*

(That equates to a yearly government savings of at least $25 million, which is spent on Alzheimer's care.)

"Estrogen reduces central obesity." *Obesity Review 2004 Nov; 5(4):197-216.*

(This in turn reduces diabetes and heart disease. The WHI trial demonstrated a 25% decrease in diabetes in estrogen users.)

"Despite popular belief that HRT causes weight gain, available data studies show no weight gain in women taking HRT compared to placebo. Prevention of weight gain is accomplished through HRT replacement, exercise and diet." *Postgraduate Medicine 2000 Sept;108(3)147-50*

(There is no magic to it.)

"The reduction in incidence of clinical ischemic events has been substantial ranging from 30% to 90%. HRT alters the biology of the vessel wall, causes vasodilation and provides anti-inflammatory benefits, reducing heart attacks." *New England Journal of Medicine 2000;343(8):572-574*

(Although the WHI showed slight harm in using estrogen in older women, all other studies show benefit. One incorrectly done study (WHI trial) does not negate 40 years of studies showing beneficial effects of HRT.

"Estrogen protects against neuron-degeneration, changes in mood, cognition and behavior." *Clinical Genetics 1998 May;6(5)15-19.*

(All of these studies demonstrate that: 1) Estradiol is safe in women who have had breast cancer, 2) Estradiol does not cause breast cancer, 3) Progesterone protects against cancer and finally.....see next study)

"Estradiol and progesterone demonstrated no increased risk of breast cancer. Synthetic estrogen (Premarin®) and synthetic progestins (medroxyprogesterone and noresterone) all dramatically increased the risk of breast cancer. This was a ten-year study of over 100,000 women, the largest and longest study to date comparing natural hormones to synthetic hormones." *Breast Cancer Res Treat 2007;101:125-134*

(Is this the final nail in the coffin for synthetic HRT? It should be!)

"The WHI trial had major design flaws that led to adverse conclusions about the positive effects of hormone therapy. The study included mostly older women that already had cardiovascular disease. The study utilized only medroxyprogesterone (Provera®) which we know negates any beneficial effect of estrogen, rather than the bio identical hormone, progesterone." Multiple other studies with estrogen started early in menopause demonstrate beneficial effects." *Fertility Sterility 2005 Dec;84(6):1589-601*

"There are now over 60 studies demonstrating that estrogen can be safely given to women after treatment for breast cancer. Most studies show a decrease in breast cancer in women on estrogen compared with controls." *Female Patient 2004 Oct;Vol 29:40-46.*

"Media reports glossed over the protection offered by HRT which showed much greater benefits than risk (remember that these are synthetic hormones). This was a classic case of hype inciting hysteria." *Female Patient 2004 Oct;Vol 29:40-46.*

"Because of the misleading reports of the WHI (Women's Health Initiative), millions of women have stopped estrogen despite the confirmed 34% decrease in hip fractures. This will result in millions more hip fractures and related deaths." *Female Patient 2004 Oct;Vol 29:40-46.*

"Because of the design flaws, the WHI trial should be discredited as it used only 2 synthetic hormones that were already known to be harmful. The positive effects of many different hormone methods studied over the last 50 years should not be discounted due to one poorly designed and flawed study (WHI) trial." *Female Patient 2004 Oct;Vol 29:40-46.*

"In the most recent, more powerful study to date, estrogen-alone (synthetic) demonstrated no increased risk of breast cancer or heart disease." *Female Patient 2004 Oct;Vol 29:40-46.*

"North American Menopausal Society (NAMS) position statement: The WHI results do not apply to the majority of women. The WHI trial does not negate 40 years of study demonstrating HRT benefit. Five recent studies demonstrate overwhelming evidence that HRT prevents atherosclerosis." *Family Practice News 2003 Oct;1-2.*

"Estrogen lowers cortisol which in turn reduces abdominal fat." *Female Patient, 2001 April; 26:18-24.*

"Estrogen therapy alters the biology of the inner vessels (of the heart). HRT protects through vasodilation, anti-inflammatory and anti-proliferative effects. HRT provides significant coronary artery benefits." *N England J Medicine 2000;343(8):572-574.*

"Estrogen protects against neuron-degeneration, changes in mood, cognition and behavior." *Clinical Genetics 1998 May;6(5):15-19*.

Progesterone

"The main reason women discontinue HRT is due to side effects. Synthetic progestins (Provera®) cause many side effects: breast swelling and tenderness, uterine bleeding, depression and mood disturbance, weight gain, bloating and edema. Natural progesterone has no side effects." *Female Patient 2001 Oct; 19-23*.

(Natural progesterone is preferential to synthetic progestins. Natural progesterone produces excellent blood levels without the unwanted side effects such as fluid retention, weight gain, breast tenderness and depression of the synthetic progestins.)

"Progesterone should be administered to all women, hysterectomy or not." *Infertility and Reproductive Medicine Clinics of North America; 1995 Oct;Vol.6(4):653-673*.

(This is another landmark study demonstrating the benefits of progesterone and the harm of synthetic progestins.)

"Due to the side effects of synthetic progestins, natural progesterone is preferred. Progesterone has proven bio-availability and no side effects making it the preferred hormone for menopause." *American Family Physicians 2000;62: 1339-46*.

(I am concerned that Provera® is still manufactured and that physicians still prescribe it and that patients still take it.)

"Synthetic progestins (medroxyprogesterone) cause depression, bloating, breast swelling, excessive bleeding, and are not tolerated by many women. Natural progesterone has none of these side effects. In fact an unexpected improvement in well-being was observed when progesterone was added to estrogen." *American Journal Obstetric Gynecology; 1999 January;180: 42-48.*

> (Still think there is no difference? Even the Ob-GYN journals mention this! Health benefits and feel-good benefits.)

"Estrogen and progesterone are neuro-protective against cerebral damage. These beneficial effects were blocked by MPA (medroxyprogesterone)." *National Academy Science USA; 2003 Sept. 2;100(8):10506-11.*

> (Progesterone protects; Provera® causes damage.)

"Natural estrogen and natural progesterone offer substantial clinical benefit over the synthetic hormones and should be the agents of choice for menopause." *Obstetrics Gynecology 1989;73:606.*

> (It has been almost 20 years since the first studies demonstrated a difference between hormones.)

"There was an unexpected feeling of well-being when progesterone was added to estrogen. Provera® decreased well-being." *American J. Obstetrics Gynecology 1999 Jan;180:42-48.*

> (Yes, there is a difference)

"Estrogen prevented cardiovascular disease. Adding medroxyprogesterone (Provera®) increased risk of cardiovascular disease and negated the beneficial effects of estrogen. Progesterone and estrogen decrease foam cell formation (plaque) whereas progestins (Provera®) increase foam cell formation (plaque)." *Circulation 1999 Dec;100:2319-25.*

(Another study demonstrating that estradiol and progesterone together protect against heart disease)

"Natural progesterone reduces hot flashes, depression, abnormal bleeding. Quality of life improves when progesterone is used over Provera®. Medroxyprogesterone (Provera®) is poorly tolerated by most women to treat PMS symptoms, fluid retention, and mood swings." _Cortland Forum, 2000 July;170-174._

> (The experts continue to say that there is no difference between natural and synthetic hormones. I wonder which drug company is paying them to say that?)

"MPA (Provera®) stimulates breast receptor sites thereby increasing breast density. Progesterone down regulates breast receptor sites thereby de-stimulating breast tissue. Natural progesterone causes no side effects." _Infertility and Reproductive Clinics of North America; 1995 Oct;6(4):653-67-70._

> (This was the first major study demonstrating the superiority of the natural hormones over the synthetic hormones.)

"Progestin, (Provera®) dramatically increases risk of breast cancer 8 times." _JAMA 2000;203:485-91._

> (This is exactly how hormones get bad press. The Media reported that progesterone causes breast cancer. This is absolutely wrong! Medroxyprogesterone causes breast cancer, not progesterone. Doctors and the media chop off the prefix _medroxy_, thereby referring to medroxyprogesterone as progesterone. Medroxyprogesterone is completely opposite of progesterone.)

"The estrogen-only arm of the WHI Trial demonstrated no increased risk of breast cancer with estrogen. This study therefore demonstrates that the breast cancer increase was due to medroxyprogesterone (Provera®) and not due to estrogen." _Family Practice News 2004 March 15;1-3._

(Isn't it amazing that when we lose a hormone that protects against breast cancer (progesterone), we replace it with a hormone that significantly increases the risk of breast cancer [medroxyprogesterone].)

(Progesterone raises good HDL cholesterol, whereas medroxyprogesterone (Provera®) lowers good cholesterol. Progesterone increases estrogen's beneficial cardiac effects, whereas medroxyprogesterone reverses estrogen's benefits. Progesterone has no side effects, whereas medroxyprogesterone has many.)

"Medroxyprogesterone stimulates proliferation of breast cells. Progesterone reduces proliferation of breast cancer cells and induces cellular apoptosis (kills) breast cancer cells."
Proturitor 2003 Dec;46(1):555-58.

(These studies should make national headlines and encourage women to demand natural progesterone.)

"The metabolic, vascular and psychiatric side effects of medroxyprogesterone can be eliminated through use of natural progesterone." _Clinical Therapy 1999 Jan;21(1):41-60._
(How could any knowledgeable doctor/patient continue to use medroxyprogesterone?)

"Medroxyprogesterone has many side effects, whereas progesterone has none." *Journal of Women's Health Gender Based Med 2000 May;9(4):381-87.*

    (There is a plethora of data and articles demonstrating the benefits of natural hormones over the synthetic hormones.)

"Progesterone reduces proliferation of breast cancer cells and induces cellular apoptosis (kills breast cancer cells) *Maturitas 2003 Dec;46(1):555-58*

    (One would think that these studies should make national headlines and make all women scramble to take progesterone.)

"Due to the side effects of synthetic progestins, natural progesterone is preferred. Progesterone has proven bioavailability and no side effects making it the preferred hormone for menopause." *American Family Physician 2000; 62:1939-46*

"Progesterone raises good HDL cholesterol, whereas MPA (Provera®) lowers good cholesterol. Progesterone increases estrogen's beneficial effects, whereas MPA reverses estrogen's benefits. Progesterone has no side effects, whereas MPA has many." *Obstetrics Gynecology 1989;73:606-611.*

    (Natural estrogen and natural progesterone offer substantial benefits over synthetic hormones and should be the agents of choice for menopause.)

"This study demonstrates that maximal reduction in breast stimulation occurs when progesterone is at its peak levels during pregnancy or late in the monthly cycle. Medroxyprogesterone increases mitotic (cancer- causing), whereas progesterone decreases mitotic activity." *Climacteric 2002 Sept; 5(3):229-35.*

(Progesterone inhibited growth of human breast cancer cells by production of certain cancer protective proteins.)

"Progesterone significantly improved quality of life over progestin (MPA). Medroxyprogesterone had many side effects, whereas progesterone has none." *J Women's Health Gender Based Med. 2000 May;9(4):381-87*

(There is a plethora of data and articles demonstrating the benefits of natural hormones over the synthetic hormones.)

"Natural progesterone, but not MPA, decreases myocardial ischemia and causes vasodilation of coronary vessels." *Journal American College of Cardiology; 2000 Dec; 36(9): 2154-2159.*

(By now one should perhaps get the impression that progesterone and medroxyprogesterone (MPA or Provera®) are the opposite of each other, and indeed they are: Progesterone decreases heart disease, MPA increases heart disease. Progesterone lowers cholesterol, MPA raises cholesterol. Progesterone prevents plaque formation; MPA increases plaque formation. Progesterone is synergistic with estrogen; MPA negates estrogen's benefits. Progesterone administration raises serum progesterone levels, while MPA has a different chemical structure that does not raise progesterone levels. Progesterone makes women feel better, whereas MPA causes depression, bloating, bleeding. Progesterone is progestational, meaning the hormone that maintains pregnancy. MPA is a teratogen that causes birth defects and is absolutely contraindicated in pregnancy. I hope I have proven my point that synthetic hormones are not the same as natural HRT.)

"Natural estradiol and progesterone are safe and show no increase in breast cancer or heart disease; however the synthetic hormones do increase risk of heart disease and cancer." *Breast Cancer Res Treat 2007 Feb 27;160-175.*

> (Although many people have an appropriate fear of HRT, this comes from media hype and the medical studies demonstrating the harm of the synthetic hormones. Do not extrapolate this to include natural hormones. This study provides credence that it is the synthetic hormones that cause the harmful effects and not the natural hormones)

"Oral natural progesterone possesses good bioavailability without the side effects of the progestins. Progestins reverse the benefits of estrogen, progesterone is synergistic with estrogen. Progestins (Provera®) increase cholesterol and lower the good HDL." *American Family Physician 2000 62:1839-46.*

"Progesterone decreases breast stimulation 400% and down regulates breast receptor sites, thereby protecting against breast stimulation." *Fertility Sterility 1998;69:963-69.*

"Mammary tumor stimulation was reduced both by progesterone and Tamoxifen, more so by progesterone than Tamoxifen, which is the drug of choice to treat cancer." *Japan Journal of Cancer Research 1985June;76:699-04.*

"Hargrove demonstrated that abnormal metabolic footprints of synthetic hormones cause harm and side effects. Serum levels of progesterone can be measured and monitored. Serum levels of medroxyprogesterone (Provera®) can't be measured as it is a completely different molecule. We and others have demonstrated that natural progesterone produces excellent blood levels without the risk of side effects of the synthetic hormones: breast swelling, fluid retention, weight gain, depression."

"Medroxyprogesterone (Provera®) up regulates (stimulates) breast receptors, increasing breast density. Progesterone down regulates breast tissue thereby de-stimulating breast tissue. Natural progesterone causes no side effects." *Infertility and Reproductive Medicine Clinics of North America, 1995 Oct;6(4):653-670.*

"Adding a progestin (Provera®) increased risk of breast cancer 29%." *J National Cancer Institute 2000;92(4):328-332.*

"Medroxyprogesterone enhances proliferation of breast cancer cells and progesterone decreased proliferation. When estrogen was added to progesterone it further reduced proliferation." *Climacteric 2003 Sept;6:221-27.*

Testosterone

"Testosterone lowers fat, improves body composition, protects against diabetes and heart disease." *International Journal of Obesity and Metabolic Disorders 1992 Dec;16(12):991-7*
(There is no medicine or therapy that protects
us as well as testosterone.)

"Loss of testosterone causes loss of libido, energy, strength, sexual function, memory, cognition, muscle and bone. Testosterone replacement, as far as quality of life is concerned, is tremendous." *Medical Crossfire 2001Jan;Vol.3 No.1:17-18*
(Thanks to medical science, we now have the
hormone that helps prevent these problems.)

"Symptoms of low testosterone may occur due to decreased serum levels or reduced receptor site sensitivity. In spite of normal blood levels patients will still feel and function better when testosterone is prescribed." *Medical Crossfire 2001 Jan;Vol.3 No. 1:17-18.*

(This is a perfect example of what most physicians do not understand. Even if a patient's hormone levels are normal, they may suffer from deficiency symptoms. This is due to receptor site resistance resulting in poor stimulation of receptor sites. This results in symptoms that can be corrected only by hormone replacement. This last statement is of extreme importance as far as symptom improvement is concerned, and this applies to all hormones. Many physicians will refuse to prescribe hormones based on normal lab values. We physicians interpret normal lab values to mean you do not need hormones. Nothing could be further from the truth. From my years of experience, the feedback from hundreds of physicians that I've trained and feedback from thousands of patients, there is overwhelming evidence that proves that patients do feel and function better when taking hormones, particularly when taking thyroid or testosterone. Don't blame your physicians for not understanding this as we are simply not trained in these concepts, even though documentation is provided throughout our medical literature.

Many physicians will inquire as to why I provide thyroid for patients when their thyroid levels are normal. They simply don't understand that optimal levels make patients feel better whereas "normal" levels do not.

This improvement in quality of life and reduction in symptoms is all due to better receptor site stimulation. Raising hormone levels to optimal levels overcomes this hormone resistance thereby allowing patients to once again feel normal; this is not achieved unless their levels are optimal.)

"Testosterone replacement improves muscle mass and strength, libido, erectile function, bone density, memory, cognition, myocardial function. It is unconscionable for physicians not to treat men with testosterone." *Medical Crossfire 2001Jan;Vol. 3 No.1:47-50.*

(Unfortunately many physicians will not treat a patient, if serum levels are normal. Testosterone as well as other hormones should be prescribed to help improve symptoms, not to treat just lab tests.)

"Low testosterone levels are associated with an increased risk of diabetes, heart disease, and carotid atherosclerosis." *Diabetes Care 2003 June;Vol. 36, No. 6: 20-30.*

(Testosterone treatment should begin at age 40 to prevent theses illnesses from progressing. Other hormones too should be prescribed to help improve symptoms, as well as preserve health and wellness.)

"Loss of testosterone causes decreased muscle mass and strength, increased fat, decreased libido, erectile dysfunction, depression, osteoporosis, decreased energy, decreased well-being, decreased protection from heart disease and bone loss. Replacement improves energy, muscle and bone strength, libido, frequency of sexual function and ejaculation. Synthetic oral testosterone raises cholesterol and lowers HDL levels. Don't confuse this with bio-identical testosterone, which lowers cholesterol and raises HDL.

Testosterone does not increase prostate volume or PSA levels or cause prostate cancer." *Archives of Family Medicine; 1999;Vol. 8:252-263.*

(Health benefits, feel-good benefits and no harm from testosterone.)

"Development of prostate cancer does not depend on levels of testosterone. High levels of testosterone do not increase risk of prostate cancer." *RR J Cancer 1999 June;80(7); 930-4*

(All medical specialty journals acknowledge that testosterone does not cause prostate cancer.)

"Testosterone levels have nothing to do with causing prostate cancer." *Cancer 1999, July 15;88(2):312-5.*

"None of the 12 longitudinal population based studies, such as the *"Physician's Health Study,"* found any increased risk of prostate cancer in men with higher levels compared to men with lower levels of testosterone." *New England Journal of Medicine 2004;350:482-92.*

(If there is anyone who still imagines that testosterone causes cancer, then they remain ignorant of the world literature.)

"Testosterone administration in the highest dosage resulted in increased sexual activity, pleasure, and orgasm in women. There was an increase in sexual fantasies, masturbation and frequency of sex. There was an improvement of well-being and mood." *New England Journal of Medicine 2000;343:682-88.*

(Theses are quotes from the most prestigious medical journal in the world.)

"Low testosterone levels increase cardiovascular disease. High testosterone levels protect against cardiovascular disease." *Diabetes Metab 1995 Vol. 21:156-161.*

(Where would you like your level to be? Remember normal is not optimal.)

"Levels of testosterone, free testosterone or DHT did not predict or cause prostate cancer." *J Natl Med Assoc Sept 2000;92(9):445-9.*

(There is no correlation between high testosterone levels and prostate cancer. Low testosterone levels correlate to a more aggressive, serious cancer.)

"Testosterone replacement in women significantly decreases carotid atherosclerosis and cardiovascular disease." *American Journal of Epidemiology 2002;155: 437-445*

(It doesn't make any difference if you are a man or a woman, both need optimal testosterone levels for cardiovascular protection and long term health.)

"Administration of testosterone to women eliminates hot flashes, lethargy, depression, incontinence, fibrocystic disease, migraine headaches, and poor libido. Testosterone also improves well-being, sexual desire, frequency and intensity of orgasm." *Consultant; 1999 August: 2006-07.*

(What more can be said? What woman would not want these benefits? Who would not want their spouse to experience these benefits?)

"Low testosterone levels adversely affect women's health. Testosterone improves women's energy and well-being. Treatment should begin when a woman's testosterone drops below mid-range of normal. Testosterone administration has many benefits and no risks. This is cutting edge work." *JAMA May 2004;Vol. 283(20): 2463-64*

(The second most prestigious journal recommends treatment with testosterone even if hormone levels are normal. They found optimum was best.)

"Low testosterone levels increase risk of diabetes and cardiovascular disease. Testosterone therapy reduces abdominal obesity, decreases risk of diabetes, dilates coronary arteries and decreases atherosclerosis." *Diabetes Care 2003;Vol. 26, No. 6:1869-73*.

(Does anyone reading this book not think that this is important? Then your doctor should also think that it is important.)

"Higher testosterone levels increase cognition and memory." *Neurology 2005 Mar. 8; 64-5:866-71*.

(And people wonder what they can do for their memory.)

"Testosterone decreases cholesterol and raises HDL." *Atherosclerosis 1996 Mar;121(1): 35-43*.

(What drugs can do this and make you feel good too? Every cardiologist should be prescribing testosterone for their patients. Do you know of any that do?)

"Testosterone improves sexual function, bone density, mood, energy, and well-being. Testosterone increases sexual gratification, desire, arousal, libido, and frequency. Quality of life is adversely affected with low testosterone." *Female Patient 2004 Nov;Vol.29:40-45*.

(That just about says it all. Even though this originated from a woman's medical journal, the same applies to men.)

"Low testosterone levels are associated with higher cardiovascular risk. Testosterone supplementation reduces abdominal fat and improves insulin sensitivity. Testosterone lowers cholesterol also." *Diabetes Metab 2004 Feb;30(1):29-34*

> (What drug does all this and makes you feel good too?)

"Hormone replacement therapy in postmenopausal women and testosterone replacement in men reduce the degree of central obesity." *Obesity Review 2004 Nov; 5(4): 197-216.*

> (Is this not healthy for us? What a shame all doctors don't recommend it.)

"High doses of synthetic, anabolic steroids cause side effects. No such side effects have been observed using low doses of natural testosterone. Avoidance of supraphysiologic levels prevents any side effects." *Female Patient 2004 Nov; Vol.29: 40-45.*

> (Many physicians and patients will remember the harm that the old, synthetic anabolic agents caused. Do not equate this with natural testosterone which has entirely opposite effects of synthetic testosterone.)

"Testosterone increases bone density in women. Testosterone protects against heart disease in women." *Journal of Reproductive Medicine 1999; 44(12):1012-20*

> (More proof that testosterone is not just a "male" hormone. It is just as much a female hormone.)

"Testosterone administration to men with PIN (pre-cancer stage) did not go on to further develop prostate cancer." *J of Urol. 2003; 170:2348-51.*

> (Testosterone administration always raises estrogen levels. Over 40 years, hundreds of studies have demonstrated raising testosterone or estrogen levels does not increase cancer. If

estrogen caused prostate cancer, as many people incorrectly and inappropriately assume, then we certainly would have observed it and we haven't.)

"Testosterone protects against Alzheimer's dementia, type II diabetes, obesity, depression, osteoporosis, muscle wasting, cognitive decline, loss of libido, erectile dysfunction, and cardiovascular disease. The prevalence of prostate cancer in men with low testosterone levels is substantial in comparison with high testosterone levels. Lower testosterone levels increase risk of prostate cancer and cancer severity.." *N Engl J Med 2004: 350: 482-92*

"Despite decades of research, there is no compelling evidence that testosterone has a causative role in prostate cancer. There is no compelling evidence at present to suggest that high testosterone levels or testosterone administration increases the risk of cancer. Prostate cancer becomes more relevant at the time of a man's life when testosterone levels decline. Experienced clinicians aim for the upper-normal range, in order to optimize treatment." *New England Journal of Medicine 2004;350:482-92*

(This was a meta-analysis or a review of many articles on testosterone. Over 40 years of articles were reviewed and there was no harm and many benefits. This was a land mark article that should dispel any fear or concern about testosterone. On the other hand it certainly establishes the harm and deterioration resulting from lack of testosterone.)

"There is no clinical evidence that testosterone replacement causes prostate cancer." *Mayo Clin Proc 2002 Jan;75:583-87.*

"Low DHT (dihydrotestosterone) predicted a higher rate of cancer. Higher DHT levels were associated with a lower risk of cancer." *Brit.J.Urol 1990 Mar;77(3)443-37.*

"Testosterone decreases visceral fat, increases insulin sensitivity, decreases blood glucose, decreases cholesterol and triglycerides, and decreases diastolic blood pressure." *Obesity Reps 1995 3:6098-6125.*

Thyroid

"Fibromyalgia is frequently seen in hypothyroidism. There is now evidence to support that fibromyalgia may be due to thyroid hormone resistance (cellular hypo-function)." *Medical Hypotheses 2003 Aug;21(2):182-89.*

> (In my experience, the most successful treatment for fibromyalgia and other body pain is testosterone and thyroid. Very few medical studies address this treatment. In this study, even though thyroid blood levels did not factor into the treatment, high doses of thyroid were used to treat symptoms.)

"Combined T4 and T3 therapy resulted in improved symptoms, well-being and weight loss in comparison with straight T4 therapy. A decrease in weight resulted from using higher T3 levels." *J Clin Endocrinol Metab 2005 May;90(5):2666-74.*

> (This is another classic article demonstrating T3 makes patients feel and function better. Physicians will continue to believe that only T4 is required, whereas the good studies in major medical journals demonstrate that adding T3 is necessary for physiologic improvement. Again this study proved as more T3 was prescribed, the better the results.)

"Long-term high doses of thyroid had no adverse effect in causing osteoporosis or fractures." *Cortland Forum July 2001:85-90*

> (Another study reviewed over 40 studies and none found any evidence that thyroid hormone has any significant effect on bone density; as these were studies of patients not on any hormone therapy except for thyroid. What this means is that the medical community cannot assert that thyroid hormone causes bone loss. Low hormone levels cause bone loss, not optimal levels.)

"TSH is a good test to diagnose hypothyroidism. However TSH is a poor measure of symptoms of metabolic severity. Therefore, it is the biological effects of thyroid hormone on the peripheral tissue, and not the TSH concentration, which reflects the clinical and metabolic effects." *British Medical Journal Feb 2003;Vol. 326:325-326*.

> (Most physicians rely only on TSH, which may result in persistent symptoms in spite of normal TSH levels. It is the level of T3 at the cellular level that is responsible for how one feels. Most physicians never measure T3 and never realize the cause of the patient's symptoms.)

"Even exceptionally high doses of thyroid do not cause osteoporosis or fractures." *Normal Metabolic. Research 1995 Nov; 27(11):503-7*.

> (Doctors are always afraid that prescribing thyroid causes osteoporosis. It doesn't and over 40 studies prove so.)

"Even though the TSH is in the normal range, patients continue to have persistent symptoms despite adequate replacement doses. These patients are still symptomatic due to low T3 levels." *BMJ Feb. 2003; Vol 326:295-296.*

"Patients that took a combination of T4 and T3 experienced better mood, energy, concentration and memory and improved well-being. Patients on just T4 experienced no change." *New England Journal of Medicine Feb. 1999;340:424-9*
(NEJM is our most prestigious medical journal.)

"Women with low-normal thyroid levels had a four-fold increased risk of heart disease. This increased risk was equal to the risk of smoking and high cholesterol. Low normal thyroid levels are a strong predictor for heart attacks." *Annals of Internal Medicine 2000; 132: 270-278.*
(Everyone would benefit from optimal thyroid replacement.)

"Low T3 levels are associated with increased heart disease and decreased cardiac function. Replacing T3 increases clinical performance and cardiac output. Adding T3 increases exercise tolerance and quality of life." *CVR & R 2002;23:20-26*

"Low levels of free T3 in patients resulted in increased disability, depression, decreased cognition, energy and increased mortality." *JAMA Dec. 2004; Vol. 292(2c): 500-504.*
(All hormones have health benefits. When we lose our hormones, we lose health benefits; thereby, increasing morbidity and mortality, and thyroid is no different. There are no studies that demonstrate optimal thyroid levels are harmful. There are many studies indicating that suboptimal or low normal levels are detrimental. Therefore our goal as physicians should be to optimize thyroid as well.)

"Low normal thyroid levels result in increased cholesterol, increased heart disease, fatigue, low energy, depression, and memory loss. Thyroid replacement eliminates these risks. No study has shown any harm or adverse effect of treatment." *Consultant 2000 Dec: 2397-2399.*

(Optimal levels are beneficial for all hormones and thyroid is no different. For healthy memory, metabolism, cholesterol, hair, skin and nails, optimal hormone levels are necessary; normal levels are detrimental.

Physicians think that thyroid administration causes osteoporosis. There are over 40 studies proving that it does not. When other HRT is prescribed, there is an increase in bone density, not a loss of bone.

Most doctors incorrectly and unfortunately prescribe only T4, whereas the studies demonstrate that adding T3 resulted in weight loss and improvement in energy and a decrease in symptoms. There was no improvement in symptoms or well-being on T4 alone (Levoxyl® or Synthroid®). Alone, or with all the other hormones, optimal levels of T3 work best.)

"Long-term thyroid replacement with high doses has no significant effect in bone density or fractures." *Lancet 1992 Jul 4; 340(8810):9-13.*

"Thyroid levels should be raised to the upper normal range for a young person. This results in optimal cognition, memory, cerebral function."
Journal of Gerontology: 1999 Vol. 54:109-115

"Combined thyroid therapy with T4 and high dose T3 resulted in improvement of symptoms and well-being, whereas straight T4 did not. Not only did they feel better, but the patients taking both T4 and T3 also lost weight. Those only taking T4 did not." *Journal of Clinical Endocrine Metabolism 2005 May; 90(5):2666-74*

"Over 40 studies prove that thyroid replacement does not lower bone density or cause increase risk of fracture." *Cortland Forum; 2001 July:85-89.*

"Decreased T3 levels result in increased cholesterol and heart disease. Treating with T3 improves the lipid profile." *Preventive Cardiol 2001;4:179-182*

Melatonin

"Melatonin has been shown to slow the growth of some cancer, prevent certain cancers, and decrease side-effects of many chemotherapeutic agents." *Medical Hypothesis 1997 June; 49(6):523-35.*

(Melatonin has become so popular that there is now a synthetic, chemically altered melatonin made by a pharmaceutical company to treat insomnia.)

"Use of melatonin in elderly patients with insomnia demonstrated improvement in sleep quality. This study is consistent with other studies." *Patient Care 2000 June:34-38.*

"In this study patients were successfully weaned from benzodiazepines (valium), with the sleep regulating hormone melatonin. Melatonin was not associated with adverse effects or tolerance." *Archive of Internal Medicine; 1999 Nov 159: 2456-2460.*

"Melatonin possesses strong antioxidant properties with increases in brain glutathione. Melatonin possesses potent anti-cancer effects, increases and improves immune defenses, inhibits tumor growth factor production." *Journal Pineal Research 1999 Aug ;23(i): 15-19.*

"Night time administration of melatonin relieves migraine headaches." *Neurology 2004 August; 246-250.*

Cancer

"Progestins increase proliferation of breast tissue. A new study shows that progesterone has the opposite effect. Progesterone was shown to not have any detrimental effect on breast tissues." *J of Steroid Biochem Mol Biol May 2005; (PubMed)*

"HRT after treatment of breast cancer has not been demonstrated to increase risk of recurrence or mortality." *J of Obstet Gynecol 2004 Jan; 23(1): 49-60.*

"Estrogen replacement therapy in breast cancer survivors results in increased survival and improved quality of life. HRT was not associated with any cancer recurrence." *Menopause 2003 Jul-Aug; 10(4): 269-270.*

"Progesterone produces breast cancer resistant protein (CRP); estrogen by itself does not. However, when estrogen is added with progesterone, the effect is synergistic by increasing the release of CRP. They are synergistic with each other." *Am J Physiol Endocrinol Metab 2005 Dec (PubMed)*

"Progesterone inhibits human breast cancer cell growth through transitional up-regulation of kinase inhibitor gene". *FEBS LETT 2005 Oct. 24; 579(25)5535-41.*

"There is growing evidence that progesterone exerts an affect on human breast tissue similar to its effect in the endometrium (protecting against cancer)." *Female Patient; Dec. 2001:3-10.*

Question: Hormone therapy and breast cancer: Does the type of progestin matter?

Answer: Yes, In this study from France of 100,000 menopausal women, the relative risk of breast cancer with estrogen-progestin regimen was 1.7%, whereas the risk for estrogen-progesterone was 1.0%. All progestins were associated with a significant increase in breast cancer whereas progesterone was neutral. The results were intriguing. This was the first epidemiologic study of this size that demonstrated no risk of breast cancer from progesterone use. All other studies, including this one, demonstrate that progestins harm breast tissue and increase cancer risk. *Breast Cancer Res. Treat. 2007; Vol.:125-134.*

(Isn't this exactly what I have preached for years? This study is exactly what is needed to silence those critics that claim there are no studies acknowledging a difference in hormone types. The *Nurse's Study* has been the largest epidemiologic study to date of 20, 000 nurses. This French study further exceeds that *Nurse's Study* by being the most powerful study to date.

Fear of breast cancer discourages many women from using menopausal hormones. This fear also fuels anxiety among physicians. However a large body of evidence from recent clinical trials indicates that the use of estrogen only therapy has no impact on the risk of breast cancer. The WHI trial, the most powerful study to date, demonstrated a decreased incidence of breast cancer. It was only through the addition of the progestin that the risk of breast cancer increased. Both patients and physicians alike should feel confident about HRT, as two very powerful studies demonstrate no increased risk of cancer with estrogen or progesterone.)

Neal Rouzier, M.D.
"The Hormone Doctor"

As a renowned innovator and leader in the field of Age Management and Preventive Medicine, Neal Rouzier, M.D. is one of the first physicians recognized for his expertise in this rapidly emerging field.

Upon completing his residency training in Family Practice and Emergency Medicine, Dr. Rouzier spent 15 years in emergency medicine in the San Gabriel Valley of Southern California. He is Board Certified in Emergency Medicine.

Dr. Rouzier has always challenged the medical field's ability to embrace the newest information. He has adapted his practices accordingly. With a commitment to transforming and finding treatments for aging, Dr. Rouzier became Medical Director of the Preventive Medicine Clinics of the Desert in 1997. Through research journals, the Internet, conferences and his private patient care, Dr. Rouzier has stayed current in age management medicine. As researchers make daily breakthroughs, Dr. Rouzier evaluates and makes available to his patients every new option.

The programs offered by Dr. Rouzier at the Preventive Medicine Clinics are the culmination of his own personal experience and ongoing research into the latest scientific studies. The Preventive Medicine Clinics specialize in the personalized evaluation and treatment of hormonal and nutritional deficiencies

His professional knowledge and teaching excellence is reflected in the popularity of his training courses. In addition to his own annually accredited CME courses, Dr. Rouzier is an invited guest speaker at various CME courses throughout the country. He is nationally sought after as a speaker and trainer. He is also the author of this successful book, _Natural Hormone Replacement for Men and Women, How to Achieve Healthy Aging._ Most important is his experience in treating thousands of patients with natural hormones.

As an avid fitness enthusiast, Dr. Rouzier exercises daily for his health and for stress relief. Along with his wife, Carolyn, he maintains a healthy diet and complete natural hormone replacement program. With the health and vitality of his 30's, Dr. Rouzier continues to enjoy his other passions, racing cars and snow skiing.

Preventive Medicine Clinics of the Desert
Director – Neal Rouzier, M.D.

2825 Tahquitz Canyon Way, Suite 200
Palm Springs, CA 92262

Office   760.320.4292
Fax   760.322.9475
www.hormonedoc.com
hormonedoc@earthlink.net

Online Resources:

My clinic web site:
www.hormonedoctor.com

Where to sign up for my live, CME accredited courses:
www.worldlinkmedical.com

Where to find a doctor in your area who has experience
prescribing hormones:
www.bioidenticalhormonedr.com

The compounding pharmacy I trust and recommend:
MedQuest Pharmacy - www.mqrx.com

A great source for nutritional supplements:
www.nutrascriptives.com

Healthy Aging blog:
www.healthyagingreview.com